Curious About Fasting?

A Comprehensive Introductory Guide to Fasting, refeeding and Sustainable Eating For Lifelong Wellness

By Dr. Jay Korsen

First Edition, 8/11/24

Table of Contents

Acknowledgements

Watching someone who you care about not eat for a prolonged period of time must be equally as challenging as actually going through a prolonged fast. Although my wife was very concerned at the start of the 14 day fast, she soon began to understand and support my journey. I could not have done it without her constant encouragement so, first and foremost, I would like to thank my loving wife who has put up with some pretty radical and unique ideas I've had over the last 40 years. Thank you Lori.

I would like to thank one of my biggest inspirations for beginning this journey, my friend Teddy Muscara. I watched him lose 100 pounds through intermittent fasting so that he was able to become eligible to receive the hip replacement he needed and he is now walking on two new hips with a transformed life because of his sticktoitiveness and commitment to accomplishing what he started. I understand now how his son Corey became so competitive and successful in baseball with a role model like his dad

I'd like to thank my friends Amanda and JP Spooner who both underwent much longer prolonged fasts than I did and provided a wealth of knowledge, tips and encouragement throughout the process.

I'd also like to thank my Chiropractic Assistant Kim who endured the ups and downs of my journey first hand at the office as I struggled to get past the challenging first few days while still seeing patients with a full schedule. Thank you also for the encouragement and cheerleading that helped me get through the finish line.

I'd like to thank my friend Gary Muniz who has also been through VERY long prolonged fasts successfully to correct serious health problems he had in the past. Your advice when I asked how I could overcome the intense feelings of wanting to eat and wanting to quit got me through the fast when you advised me to "Focus on Faith, not on feelings".

I would also like to thank my men's Bible study group whose prayers helped me accomplish my goals and reminded me that I could do ALL THINGS through Christ who strengthens me.

Introduction:

Embarking on the Fasting Journey

Welcome to a fascinating exploration of fasting! If you're picking up this book, you're likely curious about how fasting might fit into your life. As a chiropractor, I must confess that I'm not a dietician or an expert in nutrition. My expertise lies in helping people with their physical health, but my journey into fasting has been quite the adventure in itself.

My experience with fasting includes a range of methods—from juice fasting and the Gerson Therapy (which we'll dive into later) to carb-free fasting and the Daniel Fast. I even undertook a 7-day fast two decades ago. Looking back, I realize I didn't quite get it right. I broke my fast with Girl Scout cookies, and miraculously, I didn't suffer any ill effects—though I wouldn't recommend that approach!

The turning point in my fasting journey came during a 14-day water fast. On the 7th day, I found myself grappling with questions and seeking more information. I discovered that there was a significant gap in resources—a place where people like me could find comprehensive guidance not only on different fasting methods but also on the critical refeeding process and how to sustain the benefits after the fast.

Armed with curiosity and a bit of help from my trusty companion, ChatGPT, I embarked on writing this, my 11th book. While I'm proud of all my books, this one is deeply personal. It's filled with emotional experiences and lessons I've learned along my fasting journey. I wanted to share these insights in the hopes that they will guide and inspire you on your own path.

So, let's embark on this journey together, exploring the transformative world of fasting. From understanding various fasting methods to learning how to properly reintroduce foods, to choosing a sustainable life-long diet so that you can maintain the benefits of your fast, this book aims to be a comprehensive guide. Fasten your seatbelt (or perhaps loosen it, if you've just had a hearty meal), and let's dive in!

Here's to discovering the profound impact that fasting can have on our physical, mental, and spiritual well-being. Shall we get started?

What Are The Many Types of Fasting?

Fasting can be categorized based on duration, purpose, and the substances that are allowed or restricted during the fast. Here is a comprehensive list of known types of fasting:

Intermittent Fasting (IF)

1. 16/8 Method: Fast for 16 hours and eat during an 8-hour window.
2. 5:2 Diet: Eat normally for 5 days and restrict calorie intake to 500-600 calories on 2 non-consecutive days.
3. Eat-Stop-Eat: Fast for 24 hours once or twice a week.
4. Alternate-Day Fasting: Alternate between days of normal eating and days of fasting or consuming very few calories (about 500).
5. Warrior Diet: Eat small amounts of raw fruits and vegetables during the day and consume one large meal at night within a 4-hour window.
6. OMAD (One Meal a Day): Eat one meal a day within a 1-hour window and fast for the remaining 23 hours.
7. Spontaneous Meal Skipping: Skip meals occasionally when not hungry or too busy to eat.

Prolonged Fasting

8. Water Fasting: Consume only water for a set period, typically ranging from 24 hours to several days or weeks.
9. Juice Fasting: Consume only fresh fruit and vegetable juices, typically for a period of 3-10 days.
10. Dry Fasting: Abstain from both food and water for a specific period, often ranging from 12 to 24 hours or longer.

Partial Fasting

11. Daniel Fast: Based on the biblical story of Daniel, this fast involves consuming only fruits, vegetables, whole grains, nuts, seeds, and water for 21 days.
12. Calorie Restriction: Reduce daily caloric intake to a level below usual consumption while maintaining adequate nutrition.
13. Macronutrient Fasting: Restrict specific macronutrients such as fats, proteins, or carbohydrates for a set period.

Detox Fasting

14. Master Cleanse: Consume a mixture of lemon juice, maple syrup, cayenne pepper, and water for 10 days.
15. Detox Diets: Follow a diet that eliminates processed foods, sugars, and other substances considered toxins, focusing on whole, natural foods.

Religious and Spiritual Fasting

16. Ramadan Fasting: Observed by Muslims during the month of Ramadan, involving fasting from dawn to sunset.
17. Lent Fasting: Practiced by some Christians during Lent, involving giving up certain foods or meals.
18. Yom Kippur: A 25-hour fast observed by Jews during the holy day of Yom Kippur.
19. Buddhist Fasting: Often involves abstaining from food after noon.
20. Hindu Fasting: Various fasting practices, such as Ekadashi (fasting on the 11th day of the lunar cycle) or Navratri (fasting during the nine nights of Navratri).
21. Jain Fasting: Includes Paryushana (eight-day fast) and other fasting practices emphasizing non-violence and purification.

Therapeutic Fasting

22. Gerson Therapy: A dietary regimen that includes periodic fasting and detoxification practices, combined with a strict organic diet and coffee enemas.
23. Fasting Mimicking Diet: A low-calorie, high-nutrient diet designed to mimic the effects of fasting, typically followed for 5 days.

Experimental and Emerging Fasting Practices

24. Protein-Sparing Modified Fast (PSMF): A medically supervised, very low-calorie diet that provides adequate protein to preserve muscle mass while promoting fat loss.
25. Ketogenic Fasting: Combines ketogenic diet principles with intermittent fasting to promote ketosis and fat burning.
26. Alternate-Day Modified Fasting: Similar to alternate-day fasting but allows for a small amount of food on fasting days, often around 500 calories.
27. Intermittent Calorie Restriction: Alternating periods of normal caloric intake with periods of significantly reduced calorie intake.

Conclusion

Fasting encompasses a wide range of practices, each with its own set of rules, purposes, and potential benefits. Whether for health, religious, or spiritual reasons, fasting can take many forms, and choosing the right type depends on individual goals and circumstances. Understanding the variety of fasting methods available can help individuals select the most suitable approach for their needs.

The History of Fasting

Fasting has a long and varied history, rooted in religious, cultural, and political practices across different civilizations and eras. Here's a detailed look at the origins and historical significance of fasting:

Origins of Fasting

1. Ancient Civilizations:

- **Egyptians and Greeks:** In ancient Egypt, fasting was linked to religious practices and healing. The Greeks, including Hippocrates, acknowledged fasting's role in health and medical treatments.
- **Hindus and Buddhists:** In ancient India, fasting was used both as a spiritual practice and a way to achieve clarity and self-discipline.

2. Religious Foundations:

- **Judaism:** Fasting is a significant practice in Judaism, with Yom Kippur (Day of Atonement) being the most notable fast, observed with 25 hours of fasting and prayer.
- **Christianity:** Early Christians fasted regularly, and fasting practices evolved into specific observances such as Lent.
- **Islam:** Fasting during Ramadan is one of the Five Pillars of Islam, observed from dawn until sunset for a month.

Religious Reasons for Fasting

1. Jesus Christ:

- **Background:** Jesus is said to have fasted for 40 days and nights in the desert before beginning his public ministry (Matthew 4:1-2).

- **Purpose:** His fast was a time of preparation, reflection, and spiritual strength, and it emphasized the importance of reliance on God rather than physical sustenance.

**2. Muhammad:

- **Background:** The Prophet Muhammad received the first revelations of the Quran during Ramadan, a month-long fast from dawn to sunset observed by Muslims worldwide.
- **Purpose:** Fasting during Ramadan serves as a period of spiritual reflection, self-discipline, and empathy for the less fortunate. It is a means of purifying the soul and developing a closer connection to God.

**3. Buddha (Siddhartha Gautama):

- **Background:** Buddha initially practiced severe fasting and asceticism before discovering the "Middle Way," a balanced approach between self-indulgence and self-denial.
- **Purpose:** His experience with fasting highlighted the need for moderation and was crucial in shaping Buddhist teachings on achieving enlightenment through balanced living.

Political and Social Reasons for Fasting

**1. Mahatma Gandhi:

- **Background:** Gandhi used fasting as a political tool during India's struggle for independence from British rule. His fasts were both a form of protest and a means to encourage non-violent resistance.
- **Purpose:** Gandhi's fasts aimed to bring attention to social injustices, promote communal harmony, and strengthen the resolve of the Indian independence movement. His fasting also served as a personal spiritual practice and a means to demonstrate the power of non-violence.

2. **Socrates:

- **Background:** Socrates practiced fasting as part of his philosophical discipline and self-control. He used fasting to purify himself and focus his mind.
- **Purpose:** For Socrates, fasting was a way to align the body and mind, demonstrating the value of self-control and philosophical reflection.

Additional Historical Examples

1. **Plato:

- **Background:** Plato, in his works, discussed fasting as a means to achieve clarity of thought and maintain a disciplined life.
- **Purpose:** Fasting was seen as a practice to refine one's character and enhance intellectual pursuits.

2. **Early Christians:

- **Background:** Early Christians observed fasting as a form of penance and spiritual preparation. This practice was formalized into the Lenten season leading up to Easter.
- **Purpose:** The goal was to cultivate spiritual discipline, repentance, and preparation for significant religious events.

Summary

Fasting has evolved from its ancient origins as a practice for health and spiritual enlightenment to a multifaceted tradition with religious, political, and social dimensions. Its significance varies by context but commonly includes self-discipline, spiritual purification, and a way to address both personal and collective challenges. Each tradition and figure, from religious leaders like Jesus, Muhammad, and Buddha to political activists like Gandhi, has used fasting to achieve different goals, reflecting its deep and varied significance across cultures and eras.

Why Should Someone Consider Fasting?

1. Health Benefits:

- **Weight Loss:** Fasting can help reduce calorie intake and promote weight loss.
- **Improved Metabolic Health:** Enhances insulin sensitivity, reduces blood sugar levels, and can lower the risk of type 2 diabetes.
- **Cellular Repair:** Promotes autophagy, a process where the body cleans out damaged cells and regenerates new ones.
- **Reduced Inflammation:** May decrease inflammation markers, which are linked to chronic diseases.
- **Heart Health:** Can improve heart health by reducing cholesterol levels, blood pressure, and other cardiovascular risk factors.
- **Brain Health:** Supports brain function and may protect against neurodegenerative diseases.

2. Mental and Emotional Benefits:

- **Increased Mental Clarity:** Many people report improved focus and mental clarity during and after fasting.
- **Emotional Well-Being:** Fasting can help break unhealthy emotional eating patterns and provide a sense of control over eating habits.

3. Spiritual and Psychological Benefits:

- **Spiritual Growth:** Often used in religious practices for reflection and spiritual growth.
- **Self-Discipline:** Fasting can enhance self-discipline and personal resilience.

The Science Behind Fasting

1. Autophagy:

- **Definition:** Autophagy is a cellular process where cells degrade and recycle their own components.
- **Benefit:** Helps remove damaged cells and proteins, potentially reducing the risk of diseases like cancer and promoting longevity.

2. Insulin Sensitivity:

- **Mechanism:** Fasting reduces insulin levels, making the body more responsive to insulin.
- **Benefit:** Helps regulate blood sugar levels and can prevent or manage type 2 diabetes.

3. Growth Hormone Production:

- **Mechanism:** Fasting increases the secretion of human growth hormone (HGH).
- **Benefit:** Promotes fat loss, muscle gain, and overall cellular regeneration.

4. Inflammation Reduction:

- **Mechanism:** Fasting reduces oxidative stress and inflammation.
- **Benefit:** Can lower the risk of chronic diseases like heart disease, arthritis, and cancer.

Advantages of Going to a Fasting Clinic

1. Medical Supervision:

- **Safety:** Continuous monitoring by healthcare professionals ensures safety and addresses any potential complications.
- **Personalized Care:** Individualized plans based on health status and goals.

2. Structured Environment:

- **Supportive Setting:** Provides a controlled environment free from temptations and distractions.
- **Expert Guidance:** Access to nutritionists, doctors, and fasting experts for tailored advice and support.

3. Comprehensive Care:

- **Detoxification:** Facilities like True North Health Center offer comprehensive detox programs.
- **Education:** Patients learn about healthy eating and lifestyle habits to maintain after the fast.

Fasting at Home with a Consultant or Coach

1. Preparation:

- **Medical Check-Up:** Consult a healthcare professional to ensure fasting is safe for you.
- **Plan:** Develop a clear fasting plan including duration, hydration, and post-fast refeeding.

2. During the Fast:

- **Hydration:** Drink plenty of water and consider electrolytes if needed.
- **Rest:** Get ample rest and avoid strenuous activities.
- **Monitoring:** Regular check-ins with your fasting coach to monitor progress and address any issues.

3. Refeeding Phase:

- **Gradual Introduction:** Start with easily digestible foods and gradually reintroduce more complex foods.
- **Balanced Diet:** Focus on a balanced, nutrient-rich diet to maintain the benefits of fasting.

4. Consultant or Coach:

- **Expertise:** A coach trained by the True North Health Clinic can provide expert guidance and personalized support.
- **Accountability:** Regular consultations help keep you accountable and on track.
- **Education:** Learn about the principles of healthy eating and fasting to empower long-term health.

Summary

Fasting offers numerous health benefits, from weight loss and improved metabolic health to enhanced mental clarity and emotional well-being. The science behind fasting supports its effectiveness in promoting cellular repair, reducing inflammation, and improving insulin sensitivity. While going to a fasting clinic like True North Health Center provides structured support and medical supervision, fasting at home with the guidance of a trained consultant or coach can also be effective. Proper preparation, hydration, and gradual refeeding are essential for a safe and beneficial fasting experience.

Fasting vs. Cleanse vs. Detox?

In the quest for better health, many people turn to fasting, cleanses, and detox programs. These practices, while often used interchangeably, have distinct methodologies, goals, and benefits. In this chapter, we will explore what fasting, cleanses, and detoxes have in common, how they differ, and which one offers the most comprehensive benefits overall.

What They Have in Common

All three practices—fasting, cleanses, and detoxes—are rooted in the idea of giving the body a break from its usual diet to improve health and well-being. Common elements include:

1. **Rest for the Digestive System:**
   - All three practices reduce the workload on the digestive system, allowing it to rest and recover.
   - This rest period can enhance digestion and nutrient absorption once regular eating is resumed.
2. **Elimination of Toxins:**
   - Fasting, cleanses, and detoxes aim to rid the body of accumulated toxins and waste products.
   - They all promote the elimination of these substances through natural processes such as urination, bowel movements, and sweating.
3. **Improved Health and Vitality:**
   - Participants often report increased energy levels, improved mental clarity, and a general sense of well-being.
   - Each method can lead to weight loss, improved skin health, and enhanced immune function.
4. **Mental and Emotional Benefits:**
   - The discipline required for fasting, cleansing, or detoxing can foster a sense of accomplishment and control.

- Many people experience improved mood, reduced stress, and greater emotional stability.

Fasting

Definition and Types:

- Fasting involves abstaining from all or certain types of food and drink for a specific period. Common types include:
    - **Intermittent Fasting:** Alternating periods of eating and fasting, such as the 16/8 method (16 hours of fasting, 8 hours of eating).
    - **Prolonged Fasting:** Extended periods without food, typically lasting 24 hours or more.
    - **Water Fasting:** Consuming only water for a designated period.

Goals:

- Promote cellular repair and regeneration through autophagy.
- Enhance metabolic health by improving insulin sensitivity and promoting fat loss.
- Support mental clarity and emotional well-being.

Benefits:

- Significant weight loss and improved body composition.
- Enhanced insulin sensitivity and reduced risk of type 2 diabetes.
- Reduced inflammation and lower risk of chronic diseases such as heart disease and cancer.
- Potential longevity benefits due to cellular repair mechanisms.

Drawbacks:

- Can be challenging to maintain, especially for prolonged periods.
- Potential nutrient deficiencies if not properly managed.
- Risk of adverse effects such as dizziness, fatigue, and electrolyte imbalances.

Cleanses

Definition and Types:

- Cleanses typically involve consuming specific foods or beverages designed to "cleanse" the digestive system. Common types include:
    - **Juice Cleanses:** Consuming only fruit and vegetable juices for several days.
    - **Soup Cleanses:** Consuming nutrient-dense soups and broths.
    - **Smoothie Cleanses:** Consuming blended fruits and vegetables.

Goals:

- Provide the digestive system with easily digestible nutrients.
- Flood the body with vitamins, minerals, and antioxidants.
- Promote bowel regularity and digestive health.

Benefits:

- Quick and noticeable improvements in energy and skin health.
- Easy way to increase intake of fruits and vegetables.
- Can lead to short-term weight loss and improved digestion.

Drawbacks:

- Often low in protein and essential fats, which are necessary for overall health.
- May not provide enough calories or nutrients for sustained energy levels.
- Results are usually temporary unless followed by long-term dietary changes.

Detoxes

Definition and Types:

- Detox programs are designed to support the body's natural detoxification processes, often through specific diets, supplements, or treatments. Common types include:
    - **Liver Detox:** Focuses on foods and supplements that support liver function.
    - **Colon Detox:** Involves colon cleanses or high-fiber diets to promote bowel movements.
    - **Full-Body Detox:** Combines various elements such as diet, supplements, and lifestyle changes to promote overall detoxification.

Goals:

- Enhance the body's natural detoxification processes, primarily through the liver, kidneys, and colon.
- Eliminate environmental toxins, heavy metals, and other harmful substances.
- Restore balance and support overall health.

Benefits:

- Can lead to improved liver and kidney function.
- May improve skin health and reduce symptoms of fatigue and brain fog.
- Can promote weight loss and improved digestion.

Drawbacks:

- Many detox programs lack scientific backing and can be expensive.
- Some detoxes may involve harsh supplements or procedures that can be harmful.
- Results vary widely, and long-term benefits are not always guaranteed.

Comparing and Contrasting

1. **Approach:**
   - **Fasting:** Involves abstaining from food and/or drink for specific periods. Emphasizes autophagy and metabolic health.
   - **Cleanses:** Focuses on consuming specific foods or beverages to support digestion and nutrient intake. Emphasizes digestive health and nutrient infusion.
   - **Detoxes:** Uses specific diets, supplements, or treatments to support the body's detoxification processes. Emphasizes organ health and toxin elimination.
2. **Duration:**
   - **Fasting:** Can range from several hours to weeks.
   - **Cleanses:** Typically last a few days to a week.
   - **Detoxes:** Duration varies widely, from a few days to several weeks.
3. **Sustainability:**
   - **Fasting:** Intermittent fasting can be sustainable long-term, while prolonged fasting requires careful planning and supervision.
   - **Cleanses:** Generally not sustainable long-term but can be a good reset.
   - **Detoxes:** Depends on the specific program; some elements can be incorporated into a long-term healthy lifestyle.
4. **Intensity:**
   - **Fasting:** Can be intense, especially prolonged fasting.
   - **Cleanses:** Generally milder but can still be challenging due to restrictive nature.
   - **Detoxes:** Varies from mild to intense, depending on the methods used.

Which Offers the Most Benefits Overall?

Determining which method offers the most benefits depends on individual goals and circumstances:

1. **For Overall Health and Longevity:**
   - **Fasting:** Particularly intermittent fasting, offers a broad range of health benefits, including weight management, improved metabolic health, and potential longevity benefits.
2. **For Digestive Health and Nutrient Boost:**
   - **Cleanses:** Provide a concentrated intake of vitamins, minerals, and antioxidants, and can be a quick way to reset the digestive system.
3. **For Detoxification and Organ Health:**
   - **Detoxes:** Can be beneficial for supporting specific organs and eliminating toxins, though the effectiveness depends on the program's scientific backing and individual adherence.

Conclusion

Fasting, cleanses, and detoxes all offer unique benefits and can be valuable tools for improving health and well-being. Fasting, particularly intermittent fasting, is often the most sustainable and well-rounded approach, offering significant benefits for metabolic health, weight management, and longevity. Cleanses provide a short-term nutrient boost and digestive reset, while detoxes can support organ health and toxin elimination when based on sound principles. Ultimately, the best choice depends on individual health goals, preferences, and lifestyle considerations. For anyone considering these practices, consulting with healthcare professionals is advisable to ensure safety and effectiveness.

Intermittent Fasting: Types, Benefits, and Drawbacks

Intermittent fasting (IF) has gained popularity as a dietary approach that alternates between periods of eating and fasting. This method is touted for its simplicity and effectiveness in promoting weight loss, improving metabolic health, and potentially enhancing longevity. In this chapter, we will delve into the various types of intermittent fasting, analyze the pros and cons of each, and compare their benefits.

Types of Intermittent Fasting

1. **16/8 Method**
2. **5:2 Diet**
3. **Eat-Stop-Eat**
4. **Alternate-Day Fasting**
5. **Warrior Diet**
6. **OMAD (One Meal a Day)**
7. **Spontaneous Meal Skipping**

1. 16/8 Method

Description: The 16/8 method involves fasting for 16 hours each day and limiting eating to an 8-hour window. For example, one might eat from noon to 8 PM and fast from 8 PM to noon the next day.

Pros:

- **Flexibility:** Easy to integrate into daily routines.

- **Consistent Calorie Intake:** Helps regulate caloric intake without severe restriction.
- **Sustainable:** Easier to maintain long-term compared to more restrictive fasting methods.

Cons:

- **Initial Adjustment:** May require time for the body to adapt to longer fasting periods.
- **Social Constraints:** Can be challenging to fit social events and meals into the eating window.

Benefits:

- **Weight Loss:** Reduces overall calorie intake and promotes fat burning.
- **Improved Insulin Sensitivity:** Can help regulate blood sugar levels.
- **Enhanced Mental Clarity:** Many people report increased focus during fasting periods.

2. 5:2 Diet

Description: The 5:2 diet involves eating normally for five days of the week and restricting calorie intake to 500-600 calories on two non-consecutive days.

Pros:

- **Simplicity:** Easy to understand and follow.
- **Flexibility:** Allows normal eating most days of the week.

Cons:

- **Hunger:** Low-calorie days can be challenging and may lead to hunger and irritability.
- **Nutrient Intake:** Ensuring adequate nutrient intake on fasting days can be difficult.

Benefits:

- **Weight Loss:** Helps reduce overall calorie intake, promoting weight loss.
- **Metabolic Health:** May improve insulin sensitivity and reduce inflammation.
- **Adaptability:** Can be easily adjusted based on individual schedules and needs.

3. Eat-Stop-Eat

Description: Eat-Stop-Eat involves fasting for 24 hours once or twice a week. For example, you might fast from dinner one day to dinner the next day.

Pros:

- **Simplicity:** No need to count calories or worry about meal timing on non-fasting days.
- **Flexibility:** Choose fasting days based on personal schedule.

Cons:

- **Hunger and Fatigue:** 24-hour fasts can be challenging and may cause hunger and fatigue.
- **Social Constraints:** Can be difficult to participate in social meals on fasting days.

Benefits:

- **Weight Loss:** Effective for reducing calorie intake and promoting fat loss.
- **Cellular Repair:** Extended fasting periods may enhance autophagy and cellular repair.
- **Mental Resilience:** Builds mental discipline and resilience.

4. Alternate-Day Fasting

Description: Alternate-day fasting involves alternating between days of normal eating and days of fasting or consuming very few calories (about 500).

Pros:

- **Effective for Weight Loss:** Significant calorie reduction leads to weight loss.
- **Simple Pattern:** Easy to remember alternating schedule.

Cons:

- **Hunger and Irritability:** Fasting days can be difficult to manage due to hunger.
- **Sustainability:** May be hard to maintain long-term due to the frequency of fasting days.

Benefits:

- **Weight Loss:** Promotes substantial calorie deficit and weight loss.
- **Health Benefits:** May improve cardiovascular health and reduce inflammation.
- **Metabolic Flexibility:** Encourages the body to become efficient at using fat for fuel.

5. Warrior Diet

Description: The Warrior Diet involves eating small amounts of raw fruits and vegetables during the day and consuming one large meal at night, typically within a 4-hour window.

Pros:

- **Simple Guidelines:** Easy to follow once the eating pattern is established.

- **High Nutrient Intake:** Focus on nutrient-dense foods.

Cons:

- **Initial Adjustment:** Can be challenging to adjust to eating primarily in the evening.
- **Social Constraints:** Evening social activities may conflict with large meal timing.

Benefits:

- **Weight Loss:** Promotes calorie reduction and fat burning.
- **Improved Digestion:** Large evening meal may enhance digestion and nutrient absorption.
- **Increased Energy:** Some report higher energy levels during the day.

6. OMAD (One Meal a Day)

Description: OMAD involves consuming all daily calories in a single meal, typically within a 1-hour window, and fasting for the remaining 23 hours.

Pros:

- **Simplicity:** Only one meal to plan and prepare each day.
- **Effective for Weight Loss:** Significant calorie reduction due to limited eating window.

Cons:

- **Hunger and Fatigue:** Long fasting periods can cause hunger and fatigue.
- **Nutrient Intake:** Ensuring adequate nutrient intake in one meal can be challenging.

Benefits:

- **Weight Loss:** Highly effective for reducing calorie intake and promoting fat loss.
- **Autophagy:** Extended fasting period may enhance cellular repair.
- **Mental Clarity:** Some report increased mental clarity during fasting periods.

7. Spontaneous Meal Skipping

Description: Spontaneous meal skipping involves skipping meals occasionally when not hungry or too busy to eat.

Pros:

- **Flexibility:** No strict schedule to follow.
- **Natural Approach:** Aligns with natural hunger cues and busy lifestyles.

Cons:

- **Inconsistency:** Lack of structure may lead to irregular eating patterns.
- **Nutrient Intake:** Skipping meals may result in inadequate nutrient intake.

Benefits:

- **Weight Loss:** Reduces overall calorie intake.
- **Simplicity:** Easy to implement without strict rules.
- **Adaptability:** Can be adapted to individual preferences and schedules.

Comparison and Contrast of Benefits

1. Weight Loss:

- **Most Effective:** Alternate-Day Fasting, OMAD.
- **Moderate Effectiveness:** 16/8 Method, 5:2 Diet, Eat-Stop-Eat.
- **Least Structured:** Spontaneous Meal Skipping, Warrior Diet.

2. Metabolic Health:

- **Improved Insulin Sensitivity:** Most types, particularly Alternate-Day Fasting and 16/8 Method.
- **Enhanced Cellular Repair:** Longer fasting periods like Eat-Stop-Eat, Alternate-Day Fasting, and OMAD.

3. Sustainability:

- **Easiest to Maintain:** 16/8 Method, Spontaneous Meal Skipping.
- **Challenging:** Alternate-Day Fasting, OMAD.

4. Mental and Emotional Well-Being:

- **Improved Mental Clarity:** Reported in 16/8 Method, OMAD, Warrior Diet.
- **Building Mental Resilience:** Eat-Stop-Eat, Alternate-Day Fasting.

5. Social and Practical Considerations:

- **Flexible:** 16/8 Method, Spontaneous Meal Skipping, 5:2 Diet.
- **Restrictive:** OMAD, Alternate-Day Fasting.

Conclusion

Intermittent fasting offers a variety of approaches to improve health, facilitate weight loss, and enhance metabolic function. Each type of intermittent fasting has its unique benefits and drawbacks, making it important to choose a method that aligns with individual preferences, lifestyle, and health goals. Whether opting for a structured plan like the 16/8 method or the flexibility of spontaneous meal skipping, intermittent fasting can be a powerful tool for achieving and maintaining optimal health.

The Daniel Fast

The Daniel Fast is a religious partial fast based on the dietary habits of the prophet Daniel as described in the Bible. It is a plant-based diet that emphasizes whole foods and eliminates animal products, processed foods, and added sugars. The fast typically lasts for 21 days, although some variations may be shorter or longer. The Daniel Fast is often undertaken for spiritual reasons, but it also offers various health benefits.

Biblical Basis

The Daniel Fast is inspired by two specific passages in the Book of Daniel:

1. **Daniel 1:12-15:** Daniel and his friends chose to eat only vegetables and drink water for ten days instead of consuming the king's rich foods and wine. They appeared healthier and better nourished than those who ate the king's food.
2. **Daniel 10:2-3:** Daniel mourned for three weeks, during which he abstained from meat, wine, and rich foods. This 21-day period forms the basis for the typical duration of the Daniel Fast.

Dietary Guidelines

The Daniel Fast includes:

- **Fruits:** Fresh, frozen, dried, or canned (without added sugar).
- **Vegetables:** Fresh, frozen, or canned (without added salt).
- **Whole Grains:** Brown rice, oats, quinoa, barley, millet, and whole wheat.
- **Legumes:** Beans, lentils, peas, and chickpeas.
- **Nuts and Seeds:** Raw, unsalted nuts and seeds, and nut butters (without added sugars).
- **Healthy Oils:** Olive, coconut, grapeseed, peanut, sesame, and avocado oil (used sparingly).

- **Beverages:** Water, herbal teas (without sweeteners), and unsweetened plant-based milk.

The fast excludes:

- **Animal Products:** Meat, dairy, eggs, and seafood.
- **Processed Foods:** Refined grains, artificial additives, preservatives, and sweeteners.
- **Added Sugars:** Any form of added sugar, including honey and syrup.
- **Leavened Bread:** Products with yeast or baking powder.
- **Caffeinated Beverages:** Coffee, tea, soda, and energy drinks.
- **Alcohol:** All forms of alcoholic beverages.

Reasons for Undertaking the Daniel Fast

1. **Spiritual Growth:**
   - **Biblical Foundation:** Many undertake the Daniel Fast to draw closer to God, seek spiritual clarity, and practice discipline. It is often accompanied by prayer, meditation, and Bible study.
   - **Spiritual Renewal:** Fasting can lead to spiritual breakthroughs, a deeper sense of purpose, and increased faith.
2. **Health Benefits:**
   - **Detoxification:** The Daniel Fast helps eliminate processed foods and toxins, promoting overall health.
   - **Weight Loss:** The plant-based, whole-food diet can aid in weight management.
   - **Improved Digestion:** High fiber intake from fruits, vegetables, and whole grains supports digestive health.
   - **Chronic Disease Prevention:** The diet's emphasis on whole foods can help reduce the risk of chronic diseases like heart disease, diabetes, and cancer.
3. **Mental Clarity:**
   - **Focus and Concentration:** Many people report improved mental clarity and focus during the fast.

- Emotional Stability: The fast can contribute to emotional well-being and reduced stress levels.

Pros and Cons

Pros

1. **Health Benefits:**
   - **Nutrient-Dense Diet:** Emphasis on fruits, vegetables, whole grains, and legumes provides essential vitamins, minerals, and antioxidants.
   - **Heart Health:** High fiber and low saturated fat intake promote cardiovascular health.
   - **Blood Sugar Control:** The diet's low glycemic load helps stabilize blood sugar levels.
2. **Spiritual Benefits:**
   - **Enhanced Spirituality:** Fosters a deeper connection with God and spiritual renewal.
   - **Discipline and Self-Control:** Encourages discipline and self-control, which can extend to other areas of life.
3. **Mental and Emotional Well-Being:**
   - **Improved Mood:** Nutrient-rich foods and spiritual practices can enhance mood and emotional stability.
   - **Mental Clarity:** Reduced intake of processed foods and sugars can lead to increased mental clarity.
4. **Community and Support:**
   - **Group Participation:** Often undertaken in groups or communities, providing support and accountability.
   - **Shared Experience:** Fosters a sense of community and shared spiritual journey.

Cons

1. **Nutrient Deficiencies:**
   - **Protein and Vitamin B12:** The exclusion of animal products may lead to deficiencies in protein and vitamin B12 if not carefully managed.

- ○ **Calcium and Vitamin D:** Lack of dairy can result in insufficient calcium and vitamin D intake.
2. **Initial Adjustment:**
    - ○ **Detox Symptoms:** Initial detoxification can cause headaches, fatigue, and irritability.
    - ○ **Cravings:** Eliminating processed foods and sugars may lead to intense cravings and hunger.
3. **Social and Practical Challenges:**
    - ○ **Social Situations:** Dining out and social gatherings can be challenging due to dietary restrictions.
    - ○ **Meal Preparation:** Requires careful meal planning and preparation, which can be time-consuming.
4. **Sustainability:**
    - ○ **Short-Term Nature:** The fast is typically undertaken for 21 days and may not be sustainable long-term without modifications.
    - ○ **Reintroduction of Foods:** Returning to regular eating habits after the fast requires careful planning to maintain health benefits.

Conclusion

The Daniel Fast is a biblically inspired, plant-based diet that offers numerous spiritual, health, and mental benefits. While it can lead to improved health, weight loss, and spiritual growth, it also presents challenges such as nutrient deficiencies, social difficulties, and the need for careful meal planning. Undertaking the Daniel Fast requires commitment and discipline, but it can be a powerful tool for those seeking a deeper spiritual connection and improved overall well-being.

The Gerson Therapy

While the Gerson Therapy isn't a 'true' or 'strict' form of fasting, it does include periodic fasting and it's a natural treatment that activates the body's extraordinary ability to heal itself through an organic, plant-based diet, raw juices, coffee enemas, and natural supplements. Developed by Dr. Max Gerson in the early 20th century, this therapy has been used to treat cancer and other chronic diseases.

Key Components of the Gerson Therapy

1. **Diet:**
    - **Organic, Plant-Based Diet:** Focuses on consuming organically grown fruits, vegetables, and whole grains.
    - **High Potassium, Low Sodium:** Avoids added salts and focuses on foods high in potassium to balance the body's cellular environment.
    - **Specific Meals:** Includes three full vegetarian meals and up to 13 glasses of freshly prepared raw juices daily.
    - **Supplementary Foods:** Includes specific foods like oatmeal, potatoes, and vegetable soups like the Hippocrates soup.
2. **Juices:**
    - **Freshly Prepared:** Consuming 13 glasses of fresh juice daily, each 8 ounces, prepared hourly from organic fruits and vegetables.
    - **Variety:** Juices include carrot juice, apple/carrot juice, and green leaf juices to ensure a broad spectrum of nutrients.
3. **Coffee Enemas:**
    - **Detoxification:** Used to detoxify the liver and gallbladder by stimulating bile flow.
    - **Frequency:** Typically administered several times a day, with the frequency adjusted based on the patient's condition.

4. **Supplements:**
   - ○ **Natural Supplements:** Includes supplements such as potassium compound, Lugol's solution (iodine), thyroid hormone, pancreatic enzymes, and niacin (Vitamin B3).
5. **Medications:**
   - ○ **Minimal Use:** Limited to essential medications like thyroid hormone and liver extract for certain conditions.

Steps to Implement the Gerson Therapy

1. **Preparation:**
   - ○ **Consultation:** Consult with a Gerson practitioner or a healthcare provider knowledgeable in Gerson Therapy to determine if it's suitable.
   - ○ **Supplies:** Gather necessary supplies including a juicer (preferably a two-step juicer), organic fruits and vegetables, enema kits, and recommended supplements.
2. **Diet:**
   - ○ **Meals:** Prepare three vegetarian meals daily using organic produce. Incorporate large salads, baked potatoes, vegetable soups, and steamed vegetables.
   - ○ **Juices:** Drink 13 glasses of freshly pressed juice throughout the day, prepared on the hour to ensure freshness and nutrient preservation.
3. **Coffee Enemas:**
   - ○ **Preparation:** Brew organic coffee and cool to body temperature.
   - ○ **Administration:** Perform coffee enemas several times a day as prescribed, ensuring a calm and relaxed environment.
4. **Supplements and Medications:**
   - ○ **Dosage:** Take prescribed supplements and medications as directed by a Gerson practitioner.
   - ○ **Monitoring:** Regularly monitor health status and adjust supplements as needed.

5. **Support and Monitoring:**
   - ○ **Regular Check-ins:** Regularly check in with a Gerson practitioner to monitor progress and make necessary adjustments.
   - ○ **Community Support:** Join support groups or communities of individuals following the Gerson Therapy for mutual support and encouragement.

Is the Gerson Therapy a Form of Fasting?

The Gerson Therapy is not a form of fasting. While fasting involves abstaining from all or certain types of food for a period, the Gerson Therapy emphasizes a specific diet and regimen to promote healing through nutrition and detoxification. Here's how it differs from fasting:

- **Nutrient Intake:** Unlike fasting, which restricts caloric intake, the Gerson Therapy focuses on providing a high intake of nutrients through a plant-based diet and fresh juices.
- **Detoxification:** The therapy uses coffee enemas and natural supplements to detoxify the body, rather than relying on the body's natural fasting-induced detoxification processes.
- **Continuous Eating:** Patients on the Gerson Therapy consume regular meals and juices throughout the day, ensuring continuous nutrient supply and energy.

Summary

The Gerson Therapy is a comprehensive nutritional and detoxification program designed to treat chronic illnesses and cancer. It involves a strict organic, plant-based diet, frequent consumption of freshly prepared juices, coffee enemas, and natural supplements. Unlike fasting, which involves abstaining from food, the Gerson Therapy focuses on nourishing the body with nutrient-dense foods and facilitating detoxification through specific practices. For best results, it is recommended to follow the therapy under the guidance of a trained Gerson practitioner.

Why Would Someone Undergo a Prolonged Fast?

Fasting, the voluntary abstention from food, has been practiced for centuries for various reasons, including spiritual, health, and psychological benefits. While short-term or intermittent fasting (lasting from several hours to a day or two) is common and offers several benefits, prolonged fasting (abstaining from food for more than two days) provides distinct advantages that can be transformative. In this chapter, we will explore the reasons someone might choose to undergo a prolonged fast, contrasting it with the benefits and limitations of short-term fasting.

Health Benefits of Prolonged Fasting

1. **Enhanced Detoxification and Cellular Rejuvenation:**
   - **Autophagy:** While short-term fasting can initiate autophagy, prolonged fasting significantly enhances this process. Autophagy is the body's way of cleaning out damaged cells and regenerating new ones, promoting cellular repair and detoxification.
   - **Deeper Cleansing:** Prolonged fasting allows the body more time to eliminate accumulated toxins and waste products, providing a more thorough detoxification process than shorter fasts.
2. **More Effective Weight Loss and Metabolic Health:**
   - **Sustained Fat Burning:** During short-term fasting, the body primarily uses glycogen stores for energy. In prolonged fasting, once glycogen stores are depleted, the body shifts to burning fat for energy, leading to more substantial weight loss and improved body composition.

- ○ **Insulin Sensitivity:** While intermittent fasting can improve insulin sensitivity, prolonged fasting has a more profound effect, helping to regulate blood sugar levels and potentially reducing the risk of type 2 diabetes.
3. **Chronic Disease Prevention and Management:**
   - ○ **Inflammation Reduction:** Both short-term and prolonged fasting can reduce inflammation. However, prolonged fasting more effectively lowers markers of chronic inflammation, which is linked to diseases such as heart disease, cancer, and autoimmune disorders.
   - ○ **Cardiovascular Health:** Prolonged fasting can significantly improve cardiovascular health by lowering blood pressure, reducing cholesterol levels, and promoting healthier blood vessels over a longer period.

Psychological and Emotional Benefits

1. **Greater Mental Clarity and Focus:**
   - ○ **Cognitive Benefits:** While short-term fasting can enhance mental clarity, prolonged fasting often leads to more sustained and noticeable improvements in cognitive function. The brain utilizes ketones (produced during fat metabolism) more effectively, supporting mental clarity and focus.
   - ○ **Emotional Stability:** Prolonged fasting can contribute to greater emotional well-being and stability. The absence of food intake and the practice of mindfulness during fasting can lead to a more balanced emotional state over time.
2. **Breaking Food Addictions and Cravings:**
   - ○ **Resetting Taste Preferences:** Prolonged fasting can more effectively reset taste preferences, reducing cravings for unhealthy foods and promoting a preference for natural, wholesome foods.
   - ○ **Addressing Emotional Eating:** While short-term fasting can highlight emotional eating patterns, prolonged fasting provides a more extended period to address and

overcome these patterns, developing healthier coping mechanisms.

3. **Building Personal Discipline and Resilience:**
    - ○ **Mental Strength:** Undertaking a prolonged fast requires a high level of discipline and mental strength. Successfully completing a prolonged fast can enhance self-efficacy and resilience, fostering a sense of achievement and empowerment.
    - ○ **Mind-Body Connection:** Prolonged fasting allows individuals to develop a deeper connection with their bodies, becoming more attuned to hunger and satiety signals and fostering a mindful approach to eating.

Spiritual Benefits

1. **Deeper Spiritual Growth and Clarity:**
    - ○ **Enhanced Spiritual Awareness:** Prolonged fasting can lead to heightened spiritual awareness and a deeper sense of connection with the divine. By eliminating distractions and focusing on prayer, meditation, and reflection, individuals can achieve significant spiritual breakthroughs.
    - ○ **Spiritual Renewal:** Fasting for an extended period symbolizes a fresh start, allowing individuals to cleanse themselves of past wrongdoings and recommit to their spiritual path.
2. **Religious Observance:**
    - ○ **Biblical and Scriptural Examples:** Prolonged fasting aligns with the practices of spiritual leaders and figures in various religions, such as Jesus, Moses, and Elijah in the Bible, as well as practices in Islam, Hinduism, Buddhism, and other faiths.
    - ○ **Ritualistic Significance:** Prolonged fasting during specific religious periods or events holds significant ritualistic value, serving as a form of sacrifice and devotion.

Comparing Short-Term and Prolonged Fasting

1. **Health Impacts:**
   - **Short-Term Fasting:** Initiates autophagy, supports weight loss by depleting glycogen stores, improves insulin sensitivity, and reduces inflammation. However, these benefits are often moderate and temporary.
   - **Prolonged Fasting:** Deepens autophagy, promotes more substantial weight loss by sustained fat burning, significantly improves insulin sensitivity, and reduces chronic inflammation. The benefits are more pronounced and long-lasting.
2. **Psychological and Emotional Effects:**
   - **Short-Term Fasting:** Enhances mental clarity and focus, helps identify emotional eating patterns, and provides a brief reset of taste preferences. The psychological benefits are generally short-lived.
   - **Prolonged Fasting:** Leads to sustained mental clarity, addresses and overcomes emotional eating, and effectively resets taste preferences. The psychological benefits are more enduring.
3. **Spiritual Growth:**
   - **Short-Term Fasting:** Facilitates spiritual growth and renewal, offering a brief period of reflection and connection with the divine.
   - **Prolonged Fasting:** Allows for deeper spiritual growth and clarity, providing an extended period for spiritual breakthroughs and renewal.
4. **Challenges:**
   - **Short-Term Fasting:** Easier to undertake, less demanding, and presents fewer risks. Suitable for most people without significant preparation.

- ○ **Prolonged Fasting:** Requires more preparation, discipline, and medical supervision. The risks are higher, particularly concerning nutrient deficiencies and electrolyte imbalances.

Conclusion

Prolonged fasting offers a unique set of benefits that go beyond the advantages of short-term fasting. While both forms of fasting can promote health, psychological well-being, and spiritual growth, prolonged fasting provides deeper and more sustained effects. Individuals considering a prolonged fast should weigh these benefits against the challenges and potential risks, and it is advisable to seek medical supervision and support to ensure a safe and successful fasting experience.

Juice Fasting

Juice fasting is a type of fasting where an individual consumes only fruit and vegetable juices while abstaining from solid foods. This method is popular for detoxifying the body, promoting weight loss, and improving overall health by providing essential nutrients in an easily digestible form.

Key Components of Juice Fasting

1. **Fresh Juices:**
   - **Variety:** Includes a variety of fruits and vegetables such as apples, carrots, beets, cucumbers, leafy greens, and citrus fruits.
   - **Preparation:** Juices are typically made using a juicer to extract the liquid from the produce, leaving behind the pulp.
2. **Hydration:**
   - **Water and Herbal Teas:** In addition to juices, individuals are encouraged to drink plenty of water and herbal teas to stay hydrated.
3. **Duration:**
   - **Length:** Juice fasts can vary in duration, commonly ranging from a few days to several weeks, depending on individual goals and health conditions.

Health Benefits of Juice Fasting

1. **Detoxification:**
   - **Cleansing:** Helps detoxify the body by flushing out toxins and providing a break from processed foods and additives.
   - **Liver Support:** Many juices contain nutrients that support liver function and enhance the body's natural detoxification processes.
2. **Weight Loss:**

- ○ **Caloric Deficit:** By reducing caloric intake while maintaining nutrient density, juice fasting can lead to weight loss.
  - ○ **Metabolism Boost:** The high intake of vitamins and minerals can improve metabolic functions.
3. **Improved Digestion:**
  - ○ **Resting the Digestive System:** Gives the digestive system a break from processing solid foods, which can alleviate digestive issues.
4. **Nutrient Boost:**
  - ○ **Micronutrients:** Provides a concentrated dose of vitamins, minerals, and antioxidants, which can improve overall health and vitality.

"Fat, Sick and Nearly Dead" by Joe Cross

The concept of juice fasting gained significant popularity with the release of the documentary film **"Fat, Sick and Nearly Dead"** by Joe Cross.

Joe Cross's Story:

- **Background:** Joe Cross was an Australian entrepreneur who, at the age of 41, was overweight, suffering from an autoimmune disease, and relying on a cocktail of medications.
- **Decision to Juice Fast:** Seeking a way to regain his health and reduce his dependency on medications, Joe decided to embark on a 60-day juice fast, consuming only fresh fruit and vegetable juices.
- **Journey:** During his cross-country trip across the United States, he documented his experiences and shared his story with people he met along the way.

Results:

- **Weight Loss:** Joe lost a significant amount of weight (about 82 pounds) over the 60-day period.

- **Health Improvement:** His autoimmune disease symptoms greatly improved, and he was able to reduce and eventually eliminate his medication.
- **Inspiration:** The film inspired many others to try juice fasting and adopt healthier lifestyles.

Comparison: Juice Fasting vs. Water Fasting

1. Nutrient Intake:

- **Juice Fasting:** Provides a continuous supply of vitamins, minerals, and antioxidants from fruits and vegetables. This helps sustain energy levels and support bodily functions.
- **Water Fasting:** Involves consuming only water, leading to a complete absence of calorie intake and limited nutrient availability.

2. Duration and Safety:

- **Juice Fasting:** Typically safer for longer durations due to the nutrient intake, which helps prevent deficiencies and sustain bodily functions.
- **Water Fasting:** Usually shorter in duration (1-7 days) due to the risk of nutrient deficiencies and potential strain on the body.

3. Detoxification:

- **Juice Fasting:** Helps detoxify the body through the high intake of detoxifying nutrients and hydration, supporting liver and kidney function.
- **Water Fasting:** Promotes autophagy, a cellular cleansing process where the body breaks down and recycles damaged cells. This can be a powerful detox method but should be approached with caution.

4. **Ease and Accessibility:

- **Juice Fasting:** Generally easier for most people to start and maintain, as the intake of juices can help mitigate hunger and provide energy.
- **Water Fasting:** More challenging due to the absence of calories, which can lead to intense hunger, fatigue, and difficulty maintaining normal daily activities.

Summary

Juice fasting, popularized by Joe Cross's documentary "Fat, Sick and Nearly Dead," involves consuming only fruit and vegetable juices to detoxify the body, promote weight loss, and improve overall health. Cross's journey highlighted the potential health benefits of juice fasting, including significant weight loss and improved autoimmune disease symptoms. Compared to water fasting, juice fasting offers the advantage of nutrient intake, making it safer for longer durations and easier to maintain, while water fasting emphasizes deeper cellular detoxification but carries more risks and challenges.

Water Fasting
The Pros and Cons

Detailed Description of Water Fasting

Water fasting is a type of fasting in which individuals consume only water and abstain from all other foods and beverages for a specified period. This practice is often undertaken for health, religious, or spiritual reasons, and it can range in duration from 24 hours to several weeks. During a water fast, the body's metabolic processes shift to utilize stored fat for energy, which can lead to various physiological changes and health benefits.

History of Water Fasting

Water fasting has ancient roots and has been practiced by various cultures and religions throughout history:

1. Ancient Civilizations:
    - Greeks and Romans: Ancient Greek and Roman physicians, such as Hippocrates and Galen, recommended fasting for therapeutic purposes, believing it could help the body heal itself by resting the digestive system.
2. Religious Practices:
    - Judaism: Water fasting is observed during Yom Kippur, a 25-hour period of fasting and prayer for atonement.
    - Christianity: Fasting is a common practice during Lent, a period of penance and reflection. Early Christians also practiced fasting as a way to purify the body and spirit.
    - Islam: During Ramadan, Muslims fast from dawn to sunset, abstaining from food and drink, including

water. While not a pure water fast, it emphasizes the spiritual benefits of abstaining from physical nourishment.
    ○ Hinduism: Fasting is integral to many Hindu festivals and rituals, such as Ekadashi and Navratri, often involving abstinence from food and sometimes water.
3. Modern Revival:
    ○ In the 19th and 20th centuries, water fasting gained renewed interest through the work of naturopathic practitioners like Dr. Herbert Shelton and Dr. Otto Buchinger, who promoted fasting for detoxification and healing. Today, water fasting is studied and practiced in various clinical and wellness settings for its potential health benefits.

Pros and Cons of Water Fasting

Pros

1. Detoxification:
    ○ Cellular Autophagy: Fasting triggers autophagy, a process where the body breaks down and recycles damaged cells, promoting cellular repair and detoxification.
    ○ Elimination of Toxins: Without the intake of new toxins from food, the body can focus on eliminating accumulated waste products.
2. Weight Loss:
    ○ Fat Burning: As glycogen stores deplete, the body shifts to burning fat for energy, leading to weight loss.
    ○ Caloric Deficit: Consuming only water creates a significant caloric deficit, promoting rapid weight reduction.
3. Metabolic Health:
    ○ Insulin Sensitivity: Fasting can improve insulin sensitivity and help regulate blood sugar levels, potentially reducing the risk of type 2 diabetes.

- ○ **Reduced Inflammation: Fasting has been shown to reduce markers of inflammation, which is associated with various chronic diseases.**
4. **Mental Clarity and Focus:**
   - ○ **Cognitive Benefits: Many people report increased mental clarity and focus during fasting, possibly due to reduced fluctuations in blood sugar levels and the brain's use of ketones for energy.**
5. **Longevity:**
   - ○ **Lifespan Extension: Some animal studies suggest that periodic fasting may extend lifespan by promoting cellular repair and reducing oxidative stress.**

Cons

1. **Nutrient Deficiency:**
   - ○ **Lack of Nutrients: Prolonged water fasting can lead to deficiencies in essential vitamins and minerals, which can adversely affect health.**
   - ○ **Electrolyte Imbalance: Extended fasting without proper monitoring can result in electrolyte imbalances, posing serious health risks.**
2. **Muscle Loss:**
   - ○ **Protein Catabolism: Without protein intake, the body may start breaking down muscle tissue for amino acids, leading to muscle loss.**
3. **Physical Symptoms:**
   - ○ **Hunger and Fatigue: Initial days of fasting can cause intense hunger, fatigue, dizziness, and headaches as the body adjusts.**
   - ○ **Hypotension: Low blood pressure and weakness may occur due to decreased fluid and electrolyte levels.**
4. **Medical Risks:**
   - ○ **Health Conditions: Water fasting can exacerbate certain medical conditions, such as diabetes, eating disorders, and heart problems. It should be**

undertaken with caution and under medical supervision.
5. **Difficulty in Sustenance:**
   - **Mental and Social Challenges:** The psychological and social aspects of not eating can be challenging, making long-term adherence difficult.

Conclusion

Water fasting is a practice with a rich history and potential health benefits, including detoxification, weight loss, improved metabolic health, and mental clarity. However, it also comes with significant risks and drawbacks, such as nutrient deficiencies, muscle loss, and physical and psychological challenges. For those considering water fasting, it is crucial to consult with a healthcare professional, particularly for extended fasts, and to ensure it is done safely and appropriately.

Let's Be Clear, A Water Fast Is Not for Everyone

Fasting, with its profound potential for healing and rejuvenation, can be a transformative experience. However, it is vital to understand that fasting is not suitable for everyone. While many individuals can safely engage in fasting under the right conditions, there are several important contraindications that must be considered before embarking on this journey. In this chapter, we'll explore these contraindications, discuss the importance of professional supervision, and emphasize the critical role of refeeding in the fasting process.

Contraindications for Fasting

1. **Pregnancy and Breastfeeding**
   - **Why It's Contraindicated**: During pregnancy and breastfeeding, the body's nutritional needs are heightened to support both the mother and the developing baby. Fasting during these periods can deprive both mother and child of essential nutrients, leading to complications such as low birth weight, developmental issues, and reduced milk production.
   - **Explanation**: The growing fetus and the breastfeeding infant rely on the mother's nutrient stores for proper development. Fasting could potentially compromise these stores, putting both at risk.
2. **Severe Malnutrition**
   - **Why It's Contraindicated**: Individuals who are already severely malnourished lack the necessary nutrient reserves to safely undergo a fast. Fasting in such a state can exacerbate malnutrition and lead to severe health complications, including organ failure.
   - **Explanation**: Fasting relies on the body's existing nutrient reserves to sustain itself during the period of caloric

deprivation. In cases of malnutrition, these reserves are depleted, making fasting dangerous.

3. **Eating Disorders**
   - **Why It's Contraindicated**: Those with a history of eating disorders such as anorexia nervosa or bulimia may find that fasting triggers or exacerbates disordered eating patterns. Fasting can become a form of restriction, which may spiral into unhealthy behaviors and mental health crises.
   - **Explanation**: Fasting requires a healthy relationship with food, and those with eating disorders may struggle to maintain the balance necessary to fast safely.
4. **Uncontrolled Diabetes**
   - **Why It's Contraindicated**: Individuals with uncontrolled diabetes, particularly type 1 diabetes, face significant risks when fasting. Fasting can lead to dangerous fluctuations in blood sugar levels, increasing the risk of hypoglycemia (low blood sugar) or ketoacidosis, a life-threatening condition.
   - **Explanation**: Fasting alters the body's metabolism, and for those with diabetes, this can lead to unpredictable and dangerous changes in blood glucose levels.
5. **Heart Conditions**
   - **Why It's Contraindicated**: Individuals with serious heart conditions, such as congestive heart failure or severe arrhythmias, may experience complications during fasting due to changes in electrolyte balance, blood pressure, and heart function.
   - **Explanation**: Fasting can lead to shifts in electrolytes and hydration levels, which can strain the heart, particularly in those with pre-existing conditions.
6. **Chronic Kidney Disease**
   - **Why It's Contraindicated**: Fasting can lead to dehydration and increased stress on the kidneys, which is particularly dangerous for individuals with chronic kidney disease. The kidneys play a critical role in maintaining

electrolyte balance, and fasting can disrupt this, leading to further kidney damage.

- ○ **Explanation**: The kidneys are responsible for filtering waste from the blood, and fasting can alter this process, putting additional strain on already compromised kidneys.

7. **Medications Requiring Food**
   - ○ **Why It's Contraindicated**: Certain medications must be taken with food to prevent stomach irritation or to ensure proper absorption. Fasting while taking these medications can lead to gastrointestinal issues or reduced effectiveness of the medication.
   - ○ **Explanation**: Medications that irritate the stomach lining or require food for absorption can cause harm if taken on an empty stomach during a fast.

The Importance of Professional Supervision

For those considering a prolonged fast, the importance of professional supervision cannot be overstated. Fasting is a powerful tool, but it must be approached with care and knowledge. Facilities like the True North Health Center are equipped to guide individuals through the fasting process safely. These centers provide medical supervision, tailored advice, and a controlled environment, ensuring that the fast is conducted in the safest possible manner.

A fasting coach or healthcare provider experienced in fasting can assess your health, consider any contraindications, and monitor your progress throughout the fast. This supervision is especially crucial for prolonged fasts, where the body undergoes significant metabolic changes that need to be carefully managed.

The Crucial Role of Refeeding

One of the most overlooked aspects of fasting is the refeeding phase, which is the period after the fast when normal eating is gradually resumed. Refeeding is a delicate process that requires as much attention as the fast itself. If not done correctly, refeeding can lead to serious complications, such as **refeeding syndrome**, which occurs when the body is overwhelmed by a sudden influx of nutrients after a period of fasting.

Refeeding Syndrome:

- **Why It's Dangerous**: After fasting, the body's metabolic rate and enzyme activity are reduced. A sudden intake of food, especially carbohydrates, can cause rapid shifts in electrolytes, leading to severe imbalances. This can result in cardiac arrest, respiratory failure, or even death.
- **Best Practices**: Refeeding should be done gradually, starting with small, easily digestible meals that are low in carbohydrates. The process should be slow and deliberate, allowing the body time to adjust to the reintroduction of food.

Conclusion

While fasting offers numerous health benefits, it is not suitable for everyone. Understanding the contraindications and ensuring proper supervision are key to fasting safely. Whether through a healthcare provider or a specialized facility like the True North Health Center, having expert guidance can make the difference between a successful fast and a dangerous one. Additionally, never underestimate the importance of the refeeding phase; it is a critical component of fasting that demands careful attention to avoid unintended consequences. Fasting is a journey, and like any journey, it's best undertaken with preparation, guidance, and caution.

Checklist for Preparing for a Prolonged Water Fast

Before beginning my fast, I created a checklist of things to do to ensure that I was prepared and that the fast would be safe. In addition to watching every video and documentary on the subject that I could, I read books on the topic and created the following checklist which you may want to follow if you are going on this journey yourself.

1. Medical Consultation and Bloodwork

1. **Consult a Healthcare Professional:**
    - Schedule a comprehensive evaluation with a physician or a healthcare provider experienced in fasting.
    - Discuss any pre-existing health conditions, medications, and potential risks associated with prolonged fasting.
2. **Complete Bloodwork:**
    - **Baseline Blood Tests:**
        - Complete blood count (CBC)
        - Basic metabolic panel (BMP) or comprehensive metabolic panel (CMP)
        - Lipid profile
        - Liver function tests
        - Kidney function tests
        - Thyroid function tests (TSH, T3, T4)
    - **Nutrient Levels:**
        - Vitamin D, B12, folate
        - Iron, ferritin
        - Electrolytes (sodium, potassium, calcium, magnesium)

3. **Assess Fasting Suitability:**
   - Review results with your healthcare provider to ensure that you are a suitable candidate for a prolonged fast.
   - Address any necessary adjustments or preparations based on blood test findings.

2. Nutritional and Lifestyle Preparation

1. **Gradual Dietary Adjustments:**
   - **Reduce Caffeine and Alcohol:**
     - Gradually cut down on caffeine and alcohol to avoid withdrawal symptoms during the fast.
   - **Eliminate Processed Foods:**
     - Transition to a whole-foods diet rich in fruits, vegetables, lean proteins, and whole grains.
   - **Increase Water Intake:**
     - Begin drinking more water to stay hydrated and prepare your body for the fasting period.
2. **Plan the Fast Duration and Schedule:**
   - Decide on the length of the fast (e.g., 7 days, 14 days).
   - Schedule the start and end dates of the fast, and make necessary arrangements to manage your time and responsibilities during this period.
3. **Prepare Mentally and Emotionally:**
   - Educate yourself about the fasting process, including potential challenges and benefits.
   - Set clear goals and intentions for the fast.
   - Consider incorporating mindfulness practices, such as meditation or journaling, to support mental well-being.

3. Physical Preparation

1. **Monitor Physical Health:**
   - Track your weight, blood pressure, and other vital signs leading up to the fast.

o   Note any symptoms or changes in your health and discuss them with your healthcare provider.

2. **Prepare for Physical Symptoms:**
    o   Understand common fasting symptoms such as headaches, fatigue, and dizziness.
    o   Have a plan for managing these symptoms, including rest and hydration strategies.

3. **Organize Support:**
    o   Inform family, friends, or a support group about your fasting plans.
    o   Arrange for assistance or support if needed, especially if you experience any adverse effects.

4. Practical Preparations

1. **Create a Fasting Environment:**
    o   Ensure you have a comfortable and safe space to rest and relax during the fast.
    o   Prepare for possible challenges by having resources on hand, such as electrolyte supplements if needed.

2. **Set Up Hydration Supplies:**
    o   Stock up on high-quality water and consider adding mineral supplements if advised by your healthcare provider.
    o   Ensure you have a reliable water filtration system if necessary.

3. **Plan for Post-Fast Refeeding:**
    o   Research and prepare a refeeding plan to gradually reintroduce foods after the fast.
    o   Focus on easily digestible, nutrient-dense foods such as broths, soups, and soft fruits.

5. Monitoring and Evaluation

1. **Regular Monitoring:**

- ○ Check in regularly with your healthcare provider during the fast, if possible, to monitor your health and address any issues.
  - ○ Track your hydration levels, energy, and overall well-being.
2. **Post-Fast Evaluation:**
  - ○ Schedule a follow-up appointment with your healthcare provider to assess the effects of the fast.
  - ○ Repeat blood tests to evaluate changes and ensure proper recovery.
3. **Assess and Adjust:**
  - ○ Reflect on the fasting experience and any changes in health or well-being.
  - ○ Adjust future fasting plans based on the outcomes and recommendations from your healthcare provider.

By following this checklist, you can ensure a safer and more effective prolonged water fast, minimizing risks and maximizing potential benefits. Always prioritize your health and consult with professionals to tailor the fasting process to your individual needs.

14-Day Water Fast: Day-by-Day Breakdown and Tips

Day 1-3: Adaptation Phase

What to Expect:

- **Hunger:** Intense cravings for food as your body adjusts to the absence of food.
- **Energy Levels:** Low energy and potential fatigue as your body transitions.
- **Mood Swings:** Irritability and mood fluctuations due to hunger and low energy.
- **Hydration:** Increased thirst, which is normal as your body adapts.

Tips to Overcome Challenges:

- **Hydrate Well:** Drink plenty of water to stay hydrated and manage hunger.
- **Stay Occupied:** Engage in activities to keep your mind off food.
- **Gentle Exercise:** Light activities like walking can help manage mood swings and boost energy.
- **Rest:** Prioritize rest and sleep to help your body adjust to fasting.

Day 4-6: Ketosis Phase

What to Expect:

- **Ketosis:** Your body starts burning fat for energy instead of glucose, leading to symptoms of "keto flu."
- **Symptoms:** Headaches, fatigue, dizziness, and nausea are common.

- **Breath:** You might notice a distinct breath odor due to ketosis, often described as fruity or metallic.

Tips to Overcome Challenges:

- **Manage Electrolytes:** Use electrolyte supplements or add a pinch of salt to water to balance electrolytes.
- **Stay Hydrated:** Continue drinking plenty of water to support your body's functions and alleviate symptoms.
- **Rest:** Allow yourself time to rest and relax to help your body adjust to ketosis.

Day 7-10: Stabilization Phase

What to Expect:

- **Energy Levels:** Your energy levels may stabilize as your body adapts to fasting.
- **Mental Clarity:** Improved focus and mental clarity are often reported.
- **Digestive Changes:** Resting your digestive system might lead to changes in bowel movements and reduced bloating.

Tips to Overcome Challenges:

- **Mindful Eating:** Begin to prepare for refeeding by planning how you will reintroduce food.
- **Moderate Activity:** Engage in moderate physical activities like yoga or light walking to maintain health and well-being.
- **Monitor Symptoms:** Keep track of any unusual symptoms and consult a healthcare professional if necessary.

Day 11-14: Pre-Refeeding Phase

What to Expect:

- **Appetite:** You might feel an increased appetite as your body prepares to resume eating.

- **Digestive Sensitivity:** Your digestive system may be sensitive to reintroducing food.

Tips to Overcome Challenges:

- **Prepare for Refeeding:** Plan your refeeding strategy carefully to avoid digestive discomfort.
- **Hydrate:** Continue drinking water to support overall health and digestion.

Post-Fast Refeeding Period

Day 1-3: Gentle Refeeding

What to Expect:

- **Digestive Adjustment:** Your digestive system will need time to adapt to solid food.
- **Appetite Control:** You may experience heightened hunger and a need to manage portion sizes.

Tips for Refeeding:

- **Start Slowly:** Begin with easily digestible foods like broths, diluted fruit juices, and small portions of fruits and vegetables.
- **Chew Thoroughly:** Chew food well to aid digestion and prevent discomfort.
- **Monitor Reactions:** Pay attention to how your body reacts to reintroduced foods and adjust as needed.

Day 4-7: Gradual Reintroduction

What to Expect:

- **Digestive Improvement:** Gradual improvement in digestion as you reintroduce a broader range of foods.
- **Energy Levels:** Energy levels may begin to normalize as you return to a regular eating pattern.

Tips for Refeeding:

- **Balanced Meals:** Gradually incorporate a variety of whole foods, including vegetables, fruits, whole grains, and lean proteins.
- **Stay Hydrated:** Continue drinking plenty of water to support hydration and digestion.
- **Listen to Your Body:** Adjust portion sizes and food choices based on how your body responds to reintroduced foods.

General Tips for a 14-Day Water Fast and Refeeding:

1. **Preparation:**
   - **Consult a Professional:** Speak with a healthcare provider before starting a prolonged fast to ensure it's safe for you.
   - **Mental and Physical Preparation:** Reduce meal sizes and increase hydration before starting the fast.
2. **During the Fast:**
   - **Hydration:** Drink plenty of water throughout the fast to stay hydrated and support detoxification.
   - **Electrolytes:** Consider electrolyte supplements if needed to prevent imbalances.
3. **Post-Fast Refeeding:**
   - **Gradual Introduction:** Reintroduce foods gradually to allow your digestive system to adjust.
   - **Balanced Diet:** Focus on a balanced diet rich in whole foods to support overall health and recovery.

This plan outlines what to expect during a 14-day water fast and provides guidelines for a smooth transition back to regular eating. It emphasizes careful management and refeeding to support your health and well-being throughout the process.

Fasting- Refeeding After a 14 Day Fast

(Refeeding time should equal half the time the fast lasted)

Refeeding after a prolonged water fast needs to be done carefully to avoid refeeding syndrome, a potentially dangerous condition that can occur when nutrients are reintroduced too quickly after a period of fasting. The goal is to gradually reintroduce foods, starting with easily digestible, low-calorie foods, and slowly building up to more complex and calorie-dense foods. Here's a 7-day refeeding program:

Day 1

Meal 1 (7 AM):

- Small bowl of clear vegetable broth.

Meal 2 (2 PM):

- Small serving of diluted fruit juice (half juice, half water).

Day 2

Meal 1 (7 AM):

- Small bowl of clear vegetable broth.
- Small serving of unsweetened applesauce.

Meal 2 (2 PM):

- Small serving of diluted fruit juice (half juice, half water).
- Small portion of steamed vegetables (e.g., carrots, zucchini).

Day 3

Meal 1 (7 AM):

- Vegetable broth with small pieces of soft-cooked vegetables.
- Small serving of plain, unsweetened applesauce.

Meal 2 (2 PM):

- Diluted fruit juice.
- Small portion of steamed vegetables.

Day 4

Meal 1 (7 AM):

- Vegetable broth with soft-cooked vegetables.
- Small portion of plain oatmeal (made with water).

Meal 2 (2 PM):

- Small serving of diluted fruit juice.
- Steamed vegetables.
- Small portion of a baked sweet potato.

Day 5

Meal 1 (7 AM):

- Vegetable broth with vegetables.
- Plain oatmeal with a small amount of fresh fruit (e.g., berries).

Meal 2 (2 PM):

- Small serving of diluted fruit juice.

- Steamed vegetables.
- Small portion of baked sweet potato.
- Small portion of soft tofu or another easily digestible protein.

Day 6

Meal 1 (7 AM):

- Vegetable broth with vegetables.
- Oatmeal with fresh fruit.
- Small handful of nuts or seeds.

Meal 2 (2 PM):

- Steamed vegetables with a small amount of olive oil.
- Baked sweet potato.
- Small portion of soft tofu or another easily digestible protein.
- Small serving of plain yogurt or kefir.

Day 7

Meal 1 (7 AM):

- Oatmeal with fresh fruit and a small handful of nuts or seeds.
- Small portion of whole grain toast with avocado.

Meal 2 (2 PM):

- Steamed or roasted vegetables with a small amount of olive oil.
- Small serving of brown rice or quinoa.
- Portion of lean protein (e.g., chicken breast, fish, or beans).
- Small serving of plain yogurt or kefir.

Additional Tips:

1. **Hydration**: Continue to drink plenty of water throughout the day.
2. **Electrolytes**: Consider an electrolyte supplement, especially during the initial days.

3. **Portion Sizes**: Keep portions small initially and gradually increase them as your body adjusts.
4. **Monitoring**: Pay attention to how your body responds to food reintroduction and adjust as needed.
5. **Avoiding Overeating**: Eat slowly and stop when you feel satisfied, not full.
6. **Gradual Increase**: Gradually increase the complexity and quantity of food as the days progress, focusing on whole, unprocessed foods.

This refeeding program is designed to gently reintroduce nutrients and calories to the body, minimizing the risk of refeeding syndrome and promoting optimal health. Always consult with a healthcare professional before and during the refeeding process, especially after an extended fast.

My Personal 14 Day Fasting Diary

Undergoing a prolonged fast, isn't something that anyone should undertake lightly. I watched several documentaries on the subject and read several books about fasting including <u>Can Fasting Save Your Life</u> by Dr. Alan Goldhamer, DC and Dr. Toshia Meyers, PHD. Dr. Goldhamer runs the True North Health Center in California and he's one of the 'good guys' in healthcare. He was kind enough to answer many of my questions personally through email and pointed me to a plethora of resources. Before undertaking a journey into prolonged water fasting, I suggest you contact him as well.

I realized early into my fast that I was in uncharted territories so I decided to jot a few notes down for each day. I hope these notes provide some insight into what occurs in your body, mind and spirit as you go through a prolonged fast. And, although I may not have mentioned it on each day's notes, it's HARD to continue on each day. For the first few days my body begged me to quit. For the next few days my mind begged me to quit. But, I'm glad I persevered.

Day 1:
All great journeys begin with a single step. Today I took the first step towards better health. I began this journey because of an embarrassing health condition (hemorrhoids) that I was afraid was going to cause me to have surgery. Although Dr. Goldhamer was very doubtful the water fast would help, believing that the body can repair itself from anything, I'm doing this to sort of prove him wrong. I'm 194 pounds and that's down from 200 pounds just a few weeks ago using the SOS-free diet. Since I stand at 5'5" I want to be healthier and a better example for my patients. My hope is that this fast will hit the restart button for me and put me on the path to a better future.

Day 2:
I felt a little weak today. I went out for a 1 hour walk. Seems that this is easier when you're occupied by doing something to take your mind off the hunger. I've been drinking water every time that I get hungry (which is pretty often). I just want to get to bed early tonight so that I'm on day 3 soon. Everyone has told me that the third day will be the worst. Not looking forward to that at all.

Day 3:
Woke up nauseous today feeling like I have a rapid heartbeat. It feels like a fight or flight response. My mind is playing tricks on me and thinking I won't make it through the work day. I've got feelings of wanting to cut and run but I realize that this is the worst day and in the past I've taken the easy way out of things whenever there is pain or a big challenge in my life. So, I'm going to push through. I did decide not to be a 'purist' and I put a scoop of AG1 (my daily supplement) in my water. It does have 50 calories in it but I'm going to do whatever it takes to get through this and get through my day. Interestingly, the symptoms and feelings all went away after about 1 PM. I'm feeling great again. My bowel movements are really slowing down and I only went once around 2 PM. I am peeing like a racehorse however.

Day 4:
I woke up super early to go to my Bible Study this morning and I'm feeling good besides a little weakness. My chronic right shoulder pain doesn't seem to be changing with this fast but the hemorrhoids seem to be getting a little better! I decided to have the AG1 each morning but only about half a scoop which is about 25 calories. I also decided to resume taking my vitamin D and my Zinc each morning as well. It's still hard to get used to going to sleep on an empty stomach but I've found that even the mint from the toothpaste when brushing my teeth at night helps.

Day 5:
That was an extraordinarily difficult night's sleep last night. I had severe hunger pains, gurgling in my stomach, dreams of buffets and food, I was up 4 times to pee and I had pretty bad right shoulder pain. I think the pain

in my shoulder is actually a little worse. This is definitely a mental, physical and spiritual challenge/battle for sure! I was down to 183 pounds this morning from the 194 pounds I started at which is an encouragement. I had some cramping in my calf and leg today when I went for a walk during lunch. I decided to put a little Celtic sea salt in my water this evening to combat the cramps and that seems to have worked. It almost felt like 'cheating' because after the first sip which tasted like drinking ocean water, it almost began to taste like a vegetable or chicken broth. Crazy how the mind can play games with you.

Day 6:
Woke feeling a little better today. Just a little weak and shaky on rising from bed. I had a bowel movement this morning. For the life of me, I don't understand where that came from. The last time I ate was 6 days ago. I know that there are approximately 5 lbs. of bacteria in the intestines. I imagine many of them are dying off and maybe that's what created the bowel movement along with anything else being removed from my system like toxins and cells which are dying off through autophagy. I also came to an epiphany. I had such a toxic relationship with food! I was eating for comfort instead of for nourishment. I was eating emotionally instead of to feed my physical body. The mind thinks more clearly on a fast.

Day 7:
I woke today feeling abdominal gas like pain (that is beginning to 'pass' though if you catch my drift). I also still wake up a little bit weak especially compared to all the energy I had yesterday. I did take about 2 pinches of Celtic sea salt last night. Maybe that's what caused the gas pains but it seems to be completely reversing the cramping which I got in my sides last night. I took a 1 hour walk in the heat (about 90 degrees out) and there was no cramping today. Went to church today and got inspired and uplifted there to make the decision to go another 7 days to day 14. This morning I'm down to 180 pounds which is 14 pounds down in 7 days.

Day 8:

Although I had a bit of a restless sleep, I woke up not feeling the weakness or any of the dizziness that I felt the last week or so. Interestingly, I had another bowel movement last night and again, not sure how that's physiologically possible but it was small and I suppose it's from the little half scoop of AG1 I take in the morning and the cells that are being removed through autophagy. Looking forward to today and being at work where I'll have my mind occupied. Very excited about continuing to write this book. One interesting thing though, I only lost half a pound yesterday. I weighed in at 179.9 which is technically still 180 but I only write down the whole number and yesterday I was at 180.5. I suppose the weight loss will slow down a little from here on.

Day 9:
I had the deepest sleep that I've had since I started the fast and woke up rested and refreshed. I want to make a note about the extreme fatigue that happens around noon or 1PM. Apparently that's something that doesn't get described in any fasting book or documentary I watched. I consulted with my next door neighbors Amanda and Spooner who have undergone a 30 day water fast and they emphasized the importance of taking a nap or 'siesta' around that time. I'm going to try to do that and see if that solves the problem. I won't kid you, even though I'm not physically hungry, my brain keeps luring me to eat and this has become a mental battle. Besides that, everything I've read indicates that I'm getting the maximum benefits of fat breakdown and autophagy right now and it will continue until I end the fast. My weight this morning was 179 which means that I've lost another .9 pounds. I'll take that as a win.

Day 10
Although I slept great last night, I woke up with what felt like gas pains in my gut. They didn't last long but that wasn't fun. Yesterday, on my walk, I had incredible mental urges to go get food. In particular, I wanted the "junk food" like the flavored Snyder's pretzels or flavored potato chips or anything out of a highly processed, packaged bag with lots of flavor. I recognize that my body is seeking emotional comfort from them and that probably is the root cause of being overweight most of my life. Anyway, today I'm down to 178.4. Weight loss has slowed down but I'm still encouraged to see this process through. I think my biggest insight in all

this is that health and weight are not physical things, they are psychological and mental things that manifest as physical things.
Day 11
This morning two interesting things happened. First, I didn't lose any weight. I find that odd not eating but I did take about a teaspoon of Celtic sea salt in total separated out into 3 glasses of water because of spasms that I've had in my flanks and perhaps that is causing me to retain water. Two, no hunger… none. I had way more energy in the office this morning but when I got home around 2 PM I was EXHAUSTED. I took a nap from about 2:30 until roughly 3:45 and woke up only because I got a call from a patient on my cell phone. Gotta say, I do feel great. One other note is that I started this journey hoping that it would help a health condition that I mentioned earlier in this diary and unfortunately Dr. Goldhamer was right, it's not improving much. Having said that, I love the other results including clarity of thought and the spiritual benefits I've noticed being closer to God through this process. In fact, today I even gave some thought to going another week to 21 days but I think I'm going to stick to my original plan of 14 days and end this Sunday… we'll see.

Day 12
This morning was great. I woke up feeling normal, as if I wasn't even on a fast. I had plenty of energy, my mind was clear all day and we had one of our busiest days in the office which I got through with little or no fatigue. The scale went down from 177.8 yesterday to 177 which is a big encouragement to me even though I know I shouldn't use the weight on a scale to measure the many benefits to my health that a fast provides. Still, I find it an encouragement. I did discover a little 'trick' yesterday that a purest on a fast wouldn't agree with. When my mind is trying to trick me into breaking the fast, I just put a few drops of Tabasco sauce on the end of my tongue and it seems to satisfy my need to have some sort of taste in my mouth. Again, it's a mental and spiritual battle, not a physical one.

Day13
Again, I woke up feeling great. Having the scale say 176.7 was an encouragement. I only count round numbers and I'm going to use the 176 which means that I've lost 18 pounds in the last 13 days. I'll take that as a win. My energy levels are up and I'm excited to complete my last

day tomorrow and begin refeeding with a bowl of broth. Honestly, I think I could go another week but I'm more looking forward to picking an eating plan so that I can continue to lose weight consistently going forward in a more sustainable way.

Day 14
The wonderful day has arrived. I had hoped to get down to 175 pounds by the end of my 14 day fast but I'm going to have to settle for 176.1. I'll take it and I hope that I can continue to lose weight until I get down to my long term target weight of 159 after I get done with the refeeding and continued intermittent fasting for a lifetime. I feel remarkably good and, quite frankly, I'm proud of my accomplishment. It's my prayer that by having undergone this process I will be able to help others through the research I've done about fasting which I've compiled in this book. May God bless you on your own fasting journey no matter which type of fast you should choose.

40 Day Fast- Day by Day What To Expect

Make no mistake, I've never completed a 40 day fast. But, I wanted to include this chapter so that if you do try to do a fast of more than the 14 days I completed or 21 days including the refeeding period for a 14 day fast, you'll know what to expect. I highly recommend that you do not do a 40 day fast on your own without supervision from a professional trained in prolonged water fasting and refeeding.

Having said that, a 40-day fast is an extreme undertaking, especially if it involves complete abstention from food. Fasting for such an extended period can have significant effects on the body and mind. Here is a general day-by-day breakdown of what to expect, focusing on a water-only fast:

Days 1-3: Initial Adjustment

- **Hunger Pangs**: Strong feelings of hunger, which may be more psychological than physiological.
- **Energy Levels**: Initial drop in energy and potential feelings of fatigue.
- **Mental Clarity**: Possible mild headaches, irritability, and difficulty concentrating.
- **Hydration**: Increased water intake is essential to stay hydrated.

Days 4-7: Entering Ketosis

- **Ketosis**: The body begins to enter ketosis, where it starts burning fat for fuel instead of carbohydrates.

- **Hunger Reduction**: Hunger pangs often decrease as the body adjusts to ketosis.
- **Bad Breath**: Ketosis can cause bad breath due to the production of acetone.
- **Energy Fluctuations**: Energy levels may improve as the body adapts to burning fat for fuel.
- **Mental Clarity**: Possible improvement in mental clarity and focus.

Days 8-14: Deepening Ketosis

- **Stable Energy**: More stable energy levels and reduced hunger.
- **Weight Loss**: Noticeable weight loss, primarily from water weight and fat stores.
- **Digestive Changes**: Reduced bowel movements as food intake is minimal.
- **Potential Weakness**: Feelings of weakness or lightheadedness may occur.

Days 15-21: Mid-Point Challenges

- **Plateau**: Weight loss may slow down as the body adjusts.
- **Mental State**: Increased mental clarity, but potential for mood swings or emotional challenges.
- **Physical Symptoms**: Possible muscle cramps or aches due to electrolyte imbalances.
- **Hydration and Electrolytes**: Importance of maintaining hydration and electrolyte balance (consider supplementation).

Days 22-30: Sustained Fasting

- **Adaptation**: The body has largely adapted to fasting, with stable energy from fat stores.
- **Potential Risks**: Watch for signs of malnutrition or other health issues (e.g., dizziness, fainting, severe weakness).
- **Muscle Preservation**: Potential muscle loss as the body continues to use protein stores.

Days 31-40: Final Stretch

- **Severe Calorie Deficit**: Prolonged fasting increases the risk of nutrient deficiencies and health complications.
- **Close Monitoring**: Critical to be under medical supervision to monitor vital signs and overall health.
- **Physical and Mental Challenges**: Potential for severe fatigue, mental fog, and emotional swings.
- **Refeeding Syndrome**: Preparing for a safe and gradual reintroduction of food is essential to avoid refeeding syndrome.

Key Considerations:

- **Medical Supervision**: Essential throughout the fast to monitor health and prevent complications.
- **Hydration**: Consistent intake of water is crucial.
- **Electrolyte Balance**: Consider supplementation to maintain electrolyte levels.
- **Mental Health**: Be aware of potential psychological effects and seek support if needed.
- **Refeeding**: Gradual reintroduction of food is critical to avoid refeeding syndrome, which can be life-threatening.

Conclusion:

A 40-day fast is an extreme and potentially dangerous undertaking that requires careful planning, constant monitoring, and medical supervision. The effects on the body and mind can be profound, and the risks are significant. It's essential to prioritize health and safety and to seek professional guidance before attempting such a fast.

Life After A Fast- What Eating Style To Choose

Here's a comparative analysis of the Mediterranean, DASH, Plant-Based, Whole Foods, Blue Zones, Keto, and SOS-Free diets, focusing on their key elements, health benefits, and sustainability:

1. Mediterranean Diet

Key Elements:

- Fruits and Vegetables: High intake of a variety of colorful fruits and vegetables.
- Whole Grains: Emphasis on whole grains like whole wheat, barley, and brown rice.
- Healthy Fats: Use of olive oil, nuts, and seeds.
- Lean Proteins: Moderate amounts of fish and seafood, smaller servings of poultry and red meat.
- Legumes: Regular consumption.
- Herbs and Spices: Used for flavor instead of salt.

Health Benefits:

- Supports cardiovascular health and cognitive function.
- Reduces risk of chronic diseases like diabetes and cancer.
- Promotes longevity and overall well-being.

Sustainability:

- Long-Term: Easily sustainable with its variety of flavorful and healthful foods.
- Adaptability: Flexible and can be adjusted to fit personal preferences and regional availability.

2. DASH Diet (Dietary Approaches to Stop Hypertension)

Key Elements:

- Fruits and Vegetables: High intake.
- Whole Grains: Focus on whole grains.
- Lean Proteins: Includes fish, poultry, and legumes.
- Low-Fat Dairy: Recommended.
- Nuts and Seeds: Included.
- Reduced Sodium and Sugar: Limitation on added sugars and sodium.

Health Benefits:

- Effective for managing blood pressure.
- Reduces risk of heart disease and stroke.
- Supports overall health and weight management.

Sustainability:

- Long-Term: Sustainable for those managing hypertension or seeking balanced, heart-healthy nutrition.
- Adaptability: Can be tailored to individual needs and preferences.

3. Plant-Based Diet

Key Elements:

- Fruits and Vegetables: Emphasis on high intake.

- Whole Grains: Regular inclusion.
- Legumes: Key component.
- Nuts and Seeds: Included.
- Minimized Animal Products: Focus on plant sources, reducing or eliminating animal products.

Health Benefits:

- Reduces risk of chronic diseases such as heart disease, diabetes, and cancer.
- Supports weight management and digestive health.
- Promotes overall well-being through nutrient-rich foods.

Sustainability:

- Long-Term: Sustainable with careful planning, though nutrient monitoring may be needed.
- Adaptability: Can include occasional animal products for flexibility.

4. Whole Foods Diet

Key Elements:

- Whole Foods: Focus on unprocessed, natural foods.
- Lean Proteins: Includes both animal and plant-based proteins.
- Vegetables and Fruits: High intake.
- Healthy Fats: From sources like avocados, nuts, and seeds.
- Minimized Additives: Avoids added sugars, salts, and unhealthy fats.

Health Benefits:

- Promotes overall health by reducing processed food consumption.
- Aids in weight management and reduces risk of chronic diseases.

- Supports digestive health and nutrient intake.

Sustainability:

- Long-Term: Easily sustainable due to its focus on natural, whole foods.
- Adaptability: Highly flexible to personal preferences and dietary needs.

5. Blue Zones Diet

Key Elements:

- Plant-Based Foods: High intake of fruits, vegetables, whole grains, and legumes.
- Healthy Fats: Use of olive oil and nuts.
- Moderate Protein: Primarily plant sources, with occasional animal products.
- Beans and Legumes: Regularly included.
- Mindful Eating: Emphasis on moderation and mindful eating practices.

Health Benefits:

- Associated with longevity and reduced risk of age-related diseases.
- Supports overall health and well-being through a balanced, plant-based approach.
- Promotes healthy lifestyle practices.

Sustainability:

- Long-Term: Sustainable for those seeking to emulate longevity and health found in Blue Zones.
- Adaptability: Can be adjusted to fit personal dietary preferences and local food availability.

6. Keto Diet

Key Elements:

- High-Fat: Emphasis on high intake of healthy fats (e.g., avocados, nuts, oils).
- Moderate Protein: Includes meats, fish, and eggs.
- Low-Carbohydrate: Minimal intake of carbohydrates, avoiding grains, sugars, and most fruits.
- Ketosis: Aims to put the body into a state of ketosis, where it burns fat for fuel.

Health Benefits:

- Effective for weight loss and managing blood sugar levels.
- Can improve mental clarity and energy levels.
- May help in managing epilepsy and other neurological conditions.

Sustainability:

- Long-Term: Can be sustainable for those who adapt to a high-fat, low-carb lifestyle, though it may require careful planning.
- Adaptability: Less flexible due to strict carb limitations but can be adjusted for different health goals.

7. SOS-Free Diet

Key Elements:

- No Added Salt: Avoids added sodium.

- No Added Oil: Eliminates added oils and fats.
- No Added Sugar: Avoids added sugars.
- Whole Foods: Focus on whole, unprocessed plant foods.

Health Benefits:

- Reduces risk of hypertension, heart disease, and obesity.
- Promotes weight loss and overall health through clean, unprocessed foods.
- Supports digestive health and nutrient absorption.

Sustainability:

- Long-Term: Sustainable for those who can adapt to a diet without added salt, oil, or sugar.
- Adaptability: Requires careful meal planning to ensure nutritional balance.

Comparison Summary:

- Common Features: Most diets emphasize whole foods, high intake of fruits and vegetables, and balance in macronutrients. They generally focus on minimizing processed foods and unhealthy additives.
- Differences: The Mediterranean and Blue Zones diets include moderate animal products and are very adaptable, while the Plant-Based diet excludes animal products entirely. The DASH diet specifically targets blood pressure management with reduced sodium and added sugars. The Whole Foods diet emphasizes avoiding processed foods and additives but allows a variety of protein sources. The Keto diet focuses on high fat and low carbs, while the SOS-Free diet avoids added salt, oil, and sugar.

Each diet offers unique benefits and can be adapted for long-term health and sustainability based on individual needs and lifestyle preferences.

The Mediterranean Diet Pros and Cons

The Mediterranean diet is widely considered one of the healthiest diets, associated with decreased risk of various diseases (such as cardiovascular disease, certain cancers, and diabetes) and increased longevity. Here's why the Mediterranean diet stands out:

Key Features of the Mediterranean Diet:

1. **High in Fruits and Vegetables**: Emphasizes a variety of fruits and vegetables, providing essential vitamins, minerals, and antioxidants.
2. **Healthy Fats**: Uses olive oil as the primary fat source, which is rich in monounsaturated fats and has anti-inflammatory properties.
3. **Whole Grains**: Includes whole grains, which provide fiber and help maintain stable blood sugar levels.
4. **Lean Proteins**: Focuses on lean proteins such as fish and poultry, with moderate consumption of dairy and limited red meat.
5. **Nuts and Seeds**: Incorporates nuts and seeds, which are good sources of healthy fats, protein, and fiber.
6. **Moderate Wine Consumption**: Allows for moderate consumption of red wine, which has been associated with cardiovascular benefits.
7. **Limited Processed Foods**: Avoids highly processed foods and added sugars, reducing the intake of harmful additives and empty calories.

Benefits:

1. **Cardiovascular Health**: Numerous studies have shown that the Mediterranean diet significantly reduces the risk of cardiovascular diseases, including heart attacks and strokes.
2. **Cancer Prevention**: The diet's high antioxidant content from fruits, vegetables, and healthy fats helps protect against certain cancers.
3. **Diabetes Management**: Its emphasis on whole grains, fiber, and healthy fats helps manage blood sugar levels and improve insulin sensitivity.
4. **Weight Management**: The diet promotes satiety and supports healthy weight management, which is crucial for overall health.
5. **Longevity**: Populations that follow the Mediterranean diet, such as those in the Blue Zones (regions with high concentrations of centenarians), tend to have longer lifespans and healthier aging.
6. **Inflammation Reduction**: The diet's anti-inflammatory properties from healthy fats and antioxidants help reduce chronic inflammation, a key factor in many chronic diseases.

Supporting Studies and Findings:

1. **PREDIMED Study**: A landmark study showing that individuals following a Mediterranean diet had a 30% reduction in the risk of major cardiovascular events compared to those on a low-fat diet.
2. **EPIC Study**: Found that adherence to a Mediterranean diet was associated with a lower risk of cancer mortality.
3. **Meta-Analyses**: Multiple meta-analyses have confirmed the benefits of the Mediterranean diet in reducing the risk of cardiovascular diseases, certain cancers, and overall mortality.

Practical Tips:

- **Include a variety of colorful fruits and vegetables in your meals.
- **Use olive oil as your primary cooking fat.
- **Choose whole grains over refined grains.
- **Incorporate fish into your diet at least twice a week.

- **Snack on nuts and seeds in moderation.
- **Enjoy dairy products in moderation, opting for yogurt and cheese.
- **Limit red meat consumption, focusing on leaner sources of protein.
- **Enjoy meals with family and friends, emphasizing the social and enjoyable aspects of eating.

In conclusion, the Mediterranean diet's emphasis on whole foods, healthy fats, and a balanced approach to eating has been extensively researched and consistently linked to better health outcomes and increased longevity. This diet provides a sustainable and enjoyable way of eating that can lead to lasting health benefits.

Here is a 7-day meal plan for the Mediterranean diet combined with intermittent fasting, where meals are eaten at 7 AM and 2 PM. This plan includes nutrient-dense, balanced meals that emphasize whole foods typical of the Mediterranean diet.

Day 1

Breakfast (7 AM):

- Greek yogurt with mixed berries, honey, and a sprinkle of chia seeds.
- A handful of almonds.

Lunch/Dinner (2 PM):

- Grilled salmon with a lemon-garlic olive oil drizzle.
- Quinoa salad with cherry tomatoes, cucumber, red onion, and feta cheese.
- Steamed broccoli.

Day 2

Breakfast (7 AM):

- Overnight oats made with oats, almond milk, walnuts, and a dash of cinnamon, topped with fresh sliced banana.
- Green tea.

Lunch/Dinner (2 PM):

- Mediterranean chickpea salad with cucumbers, tomatoes, red onion, Kalamata olives, and parsley, dressed with olive oil and lemon juice.
- Whole grain pita bread.
- Sliced avocado.

Day 3

Breakfast (7 AM):

- Whole grain toast with mashed avocado, a poached egg, and a sprinkle of red pepper flakes.
- A small apple.

Lunch/Dinner (2 PM):

- Baked chicken breast with rosemary and garlic.
- Roasted sweet potatoes.
- Mixed greens salad with olive oil and balsamic vinegar.

Day 4

Breakfast (7 AM):

- Smoothie with spinach, frozen berries, Greek yogurt, flax seeds, and almond milk.
- A small handful of walnuts.

Lunch/Dinner (2 PM):

- Tuna salad made with olive oil, lemon juice, celery, red onion, and mixed greens.
- Whole grain crackers.
- A side of cherry tomatoes.

Day 5

Breakfast (7 AM):

- Scrambled eggs with spinach, tomatoes, and feta cheese.
- Whole grain toast.
- A small orange.

Lunch/Dinner (2 PM):

- Stuffed bell peppers with quinoa, black beans, corn, tomatoes, and spices, topped with a bit of shredded cheese.
- A side of mixed greens with olive oil and vinegar.

Day 6

Breakfast (7 AM):

- Greek yogurt parfait with granola, fresh strawberries, and a drizzle of honey.
- A small handful of pistachios.

Lunch/Dinner (2 PM):

- Grilled shrimp with garlic and lemon.
- Brown rice pilaf with vegetables.
- Steamed asparagus.

Day 7

Breakfast (7 AM):

- Whole grain waffle topped with fresh berries and a dollop of Greek yogurt.
- Green tea.

Lunch/Dinner (2 PM):

- Eggplant parmesan made with baked eggplant slices, marinara sauce, and a light sprinkle of mozzarella cheese.
- Whole grain pasta.
- A side salad with mixed greens, tomatoes, cucumber, and olive oil dressing.

Tips for the Mediterranean Diet and Intermittent Fasting:

1. **Hydration**: Drink plenty of water throughout the day, especially between fasting periods.
2. **Healthy Fats**: Incorporate sources of healthy fats such as olive oil, avocados, nuts, and seeds.
3. **Whole Grains**: Choose whole grains like quinoa, brown rice, and whole grain bread and pasta.
4. **Lean Proteins**: Focus on lean proteins like fish, chicken, legumes, and Greek yogurt.
5. **Fruits and Vegetables**: Include a variety of colorful fruits and vegetables in your meals.
6. **Herbs and Spices**: Use herbs and spices to enhance flavor without adding salt.

This meal plan balances nutrient-dense foods with the principles of the Mediterranean diet, making it suitable for someone practicing intermittent fasting with two meals a day.

The Blue Zones Diet Pros and Cons

Pros:

1. **Longevity and Health:**
   - **Increased Lifespan:** Associated with longer life expectancy and reduced incidence of age-related diseases.
   - **Reduced Chronic Disease:** Lowers the risk of heart disease, cancer, and diabetes.
2. **Balanced Nutrition:**
   - **Plant-Based Emphasis:** High intake of fruits, vegetables, legumes, and whole grains supports overall health.
   - **Healthy Fats:** Use of olive oil and nuts contributes to heart health.
   - **Moderate Protein:** Primarily from plant sources, with occasional animal products, supports muscle health without excess.
3. **Lifestyle Factors:**
   - **Community and Purpose:** Emphasizes social connections and a sense of purpose, which are linked to better mental and emotional health.
   - **Physical Activity:** Regular, moderate exercise is a part of daily life.
4. **Mindful Eating:**
   - **Portion Control:** Encourages moderate eating and mindful consumption, which can prevent overeating.

Cons:

1. **Limited Animal Products:**

- o **Protein Sources:** Animal products are consumed only occasionally, which may be a challenge for those needing higher protein intake.
  - o **Variety:** Less emphasis on animal-based options may not suit everyone's dietary preferences.
2. **Social and Cultural Adaptation:**
   - o **Dietary Changes:** Adjusting to a Blue Zones diet may require significant changes for those accustomed to a more conventional diet.
   - o **Availability:** Access to certain Blue Zones-specific foods may be limited depending on location.
3. **Nutrient Monitoring:**
   - o **Potential Deficiencies:** While generally nutrient-dense, some individuals may need to ensure they get adequate amounts of certain nutrients, like vitamin B12, if animal products are minimal.

Long-Term Successes and Health Outcomes

1. Longevity:

- **Extended Lifespan:** Populations in Blue Zones are known for their remarkable longevity, often living to 100 years or more.

2. Chronic Disease Prevention:

- **Reduced Incidence:** Lower rates of cardiovascular diseases, cancers, and type 2 diabetes among Blue Zones populations.

3. Quality of Life:

- **Healthy Aging:** Individuals maintain good health and functional independence into old age.

4. Mental and Emotional Well-Being:

- **Social Engagement:** Strong community ties and a sense of purpose contribute to mental well-being and reduce stress levels.

7-Day Blue Zones Meal Plan with Intermittent Fasting

Day 1

- **7 AM:** Oatmeal with fresh berries, a tablespoon of chia seeds, and a sprinkle of cinnamon.
- **2 PM:** Lentil stew with carrots, celery, tomatoes, and a side of mixed greens salad with a lemon-olive oil dressing.

Day 2

- **7 AM:** Smoothie with spinach, banana, frozen berries, flaxseeds, and unsweetened almond milk.
- **2 PM:** Quinoa and chickpea salad with cucumbers, bell peppers, cherry tomatoes, and a balsamic vinaigrette.

Day 3

- **7 AM:** Whole grain toast with avocado and tomato slices, and a side of fruit (e.g., an apple).
- **2 PM:** Stuffed bell peppers with brown rice, black beans, corn, and a side of steamed broccoli.

Day 4

- **7 AM:** Greek yogurt with a mix of nuts and seeds and a drizzle of honey.
- **2 PM:** Vegetable and bean soup with a side of whole grain bread.

Day 5

- **7 AM:** Chia pudding made with coconut milk, topped with kiwi and strawberries.
- **2 PM:** Sweet potato and black bean tacos with avocado, salsa, and a side of mixed greens.

Day 6

- **7 AM:** Buckwheat pancakes topped with fresh blueberries and a handful of walnuts.
- **2 PM:** Baked falafel with a side of tabbouleh salad and hummus.

Day 7

- **7 AM:** Fruit smoothie bowl with blended mango, spinach, and almond milk, topped with granola and fresh berries.
- **2 PM:** Roasted vegetable medley (carrots, zucchini, bell peppers) with a side of quinoa.

Additional Tips:

- **Hydration:** Drink plenty of water throughout the day.
- **Nutrient Diversity:** Ensure a wide range of vegetables, fruits, legumes, and whole grains for balanced nutrition.
- **Mindful Eating:** Pay attention to portion sizes and eat slowly to support digestive health.

This meal plan incorporates the principles of the Blue Zones diet with intermittent fasting, focusing on nutrient-dense, plant-based foods and mindful eating practices.

The Plant-Based Diet Pros and Cons

Pros:

1. **Improved Heart Health:**
   - **Reduced Risk of Cardiovascular Disease:** Plant-based diets are low in saturated fats and cholesterol, which can help lower blood pressure and cholesterol levels, reducing the risk of heart disease.
   - **Anti-Inflammatory:** Rich in antioxidants and anti-inflammatory compounds from fruits, vegetables, nuts, and seeds.
2. **Better Weight Management:**
   - **Lower Caloric Density:** Plant-based foods are generally lower in calories and higher in fiber, which can aid in weight loss and weight maintenance.
   - **Increased Satiety:** High fiber content helps in feeling fuller longer.
3. **Lower Risk of Chronic Diseases:**
   - **Diabetes:** Can improve insulin sensitivity and lower the risk of type 2 diabetes.
   - **Cancer:** Some studies suggest a lower risk of certain types of cancer, such as colorectal cancer.
4. **Enhanced Digestive Health:**
   - **High Fiber Content:** Promotes regular bowel movements and supports a healthy gut microbiome.
5. **Environmental Benefits:**
   - **Sustainability:** Lower carbon footprint and reduced environmental impact compared to diets high in animal products.

Cons:

1. **Potential Nutrient Deficiencies:**
   - **Vitamin B12:** Essential for nerve function and blood formation; primarily found in animal products. Supplementation may be necessary.
   - **Iron and Zinc:** Plant-based sources of iron and zinc are less easily absorbed than those from animal products.
   - **Omega-3 Fatty Acids:** May require sources like flaxseeds or algae supplements to meet needs.
2. **Social and Cultural Challenges:**
   - **Limited Options:** May face difficulties finding suitable options when dining out or attending social gatherings.
   - **Perceived Lack of Variety:** Some people may find plant-based diets less satisfying if they are not familiar with diverse plant-based foods.
3. **Initial Adjustment Period:**
   - **Adaptation:** Transitioning to a plant-based diet can be challenging and may require careful planning to ensure balanced nutrition.

Long-Term Successes and Health Outcomes

1. Weight Management and Obesity Prevention:

- **Studies:** Plant-based diets have been associated with lower body mass index (BMI) and reduced risk of obesity.

2. Cardiovascular Health:

- **Research:** Long-term adherence to plant-based diets is linked with lower cholesterol levels, reduced blood pressure, and a lower incidence of heart disease.

3. Diabetes Management:

- **Evidence:** Improved glycemic control and reduced risk of developing type 2 diabetes are commonly reported among those on plant-based diets.

4. Cancer Prevention:

- **Findings:** Some research suggests a lower risk of certain cancers, though results can vary depending on the specific type of cancer.

5. Longevity:

- **Studies:** Populations with predominantly plant-based diets, such as those in Blue Zones, often exhibit longer lifespans and lower rates of age-related diseases.

7-Day Plant-Based Meal Plan with Intermittent Fasting

Day 1

- **7 AM:** Smoothie with spinach, banana, frozen berries, flaxseeds, and unsweetened almond milk.
- **2 PM:** Quinoa salad with chickpeas, cucumber, cherry tomatoes, bell pepper, and a lemon-tahini dressing.

Day 2

- **7 AM:** Overnight oats with chia seeds, almond milk, sliced apples, and a sprinkle of cinnamon.
- **2 PM:** Lentil soup with carrots, celery, onions, and kale. Side of steamed broccoli.

Day 3

- **7 AM:** Whole grain toast with avocado, tomato slices, and a side of fresh fruit (such as berries).
- **2 PM:** Brown rice and black bean bowl with corn, diced tomatoes, avocado, and cilantro.

Day 4

- **7 AM:** Chia pudding made with coconut milk and topped with kiwi and strawberries.
- **2 PM:** Stuffed bell peppers with quinoa, spinach, black beans, and a side of mixed greens salad.

Day 5

- **7 AM:** Fruit salad with a variety of seasonal fruits and a handful of raw walnuts.
- **2 PM:** Sweet potato and black bean chili with diced tomatoes, corn, and bell peppers.

Day 6

- **7 AM:** Smoothie bowl with blended banana, spinach, and almond milk, topped with granola and fresh berries.
- **2 PM:** Stir-fried tofu with mixed vegetables (bell peppers, broccoli, snap peas) over brown rice.

Day 7

- **7 AM:** Buckwheat porridge with almond milk, topped with sliced banana and a sprinkle of chia seeds.
- **2 PM:** Chickpea and vegetable curry with cauliflower rice.

Additional Tips:

- **Hydration:** Drink plenty of water throughout the day.
- **Nutrient Balancing:** Ensure variety in food choices to cover essential nutrients.
- **Meal Prep:** Prepare meals in advance to make sticking to the plan easier.

This meal plan provides a balanced and nutrient-dense approach to combining a plant-based diet with intermittent fasting.

SOS-Free Diet Pros and Cons

The Salt, Oil, and Sugar-Free (SOS-Free) diet is a plant-based dietary approach that eliminates added salt, oil, and sugar. Advocates of this diet argue that it promotes optimal health by reducing the risk of chronic diseases and encouraging the consumption of whole, unprocessed foods. Here are the pros and cons of the SOS-Free diet:

Pros of the SOS-Free Diet:

1. **Reduction in Processed Foods**: By eliminating added salt, oil, and sugar, the diet naturally reduces the intake of processed and packaged foods, which are often high in unhealthy additives.
2. **Improved Heart Health**: Reducing salt intake can lower blood pressure, while avoiding oils can decrease the intake of unhealthy fats. Both factors contribute to better cardiovascular health.
3. **Weight Management**: Without added sugars and oils, the diet can help reduce calorie intake, promoting weight loss and maintenance of a healthy weight.
4. **Lower Risk of Chronic Diseases**: High consumption of added sugars, oils, and salt is linked to various chronic diseases, including heart disease, diabetes, and hypertension. The SOS-Free diet aims to minimize these risks.
5. **Enhanced Nutrient Intake**: The diet emphasizes whole, plant-based foods, which are rich in essential nutrients, fiber, vitamins, and minerals.
6. **Reduced Inflammation**: By focusing on whole foods and avoiding processed ingredients, the diet may help reduce systemic inflammation, a contributor to many chronic conditions.

Cons of the SOS-Free Diet:

1. **Difficulty in Adherence**: The diet's restrictive nature can make it challenging to maintain, especially in social situations or when dining out.
2. **Potential Nutrient Deficiencies**: Completely eliminating oil can result in a lack of essential fatty acids. It's important to ensure adequate intake of healthy fats from whole food sources like nuts, seeds, and avocados.
3. **Limited Flavor**: Removing added salt, oil, and sugar can make food taste bland, which may reduce enjoyment and satisfaction with meals.
4. **Cooking Challenges**: Cooking without oil can be difficult, as oil is often used for sautéing, baking, and adding texture and flavor to dishes.
5. **Lack of Flexibility**: The diet's strict guidelines can be difficult to follow long-term, potentially leading to feelings of deprivation or frustration.
6. **Social and Cultural Impact**: Food plays a significant role in social and cultural settings. The restrictions of the SOS-Free diet can make it harder to participate in social gatherings and enjoy traditional foods.

Practical Tips for Following an SOS-Free Diet:

- **Use Herbs and Spices**: Enhance flavor with a variety of herbs, spices, and aromatic vegetables like garlic and onions.
- **Focus on Whole Foods**: Prioritize whole grains, legumes, fruits, vegetables, nuts, and seeds to ensure a balanced and nutrient-dense diet.
- **Healthy Fats**: Obtain essential fatty acids from whole food sources such as flaxseeds, chia seeds, walnuts, and avocados.
- **Cooking Methods**: Experiment with cooking methods that don't require oil, such as steaming, boiling, baking, and using non-stick cookware or water sautéing.
- **Read Labels**: Be vigilant about reading food labels to avoid hidden sources of salt, oil, and sugar in packaged foods.

- **Plan Ahead**: Prepare meals in advance and carry SOS-Free
  snacks to stay on track when away from home.

Conclusion:

The SOS-Free diet can offer significant health benefits by reducing the
intake of processed foods and focusing on whole, nutrient-dense plant-
based foods. However, it also poses challenges in terms of adherence,
flavor, and social interactions. It is essential to approach this diet with
careful planning and consideration of potential nutrient needs to ensure it
is sustainable and enjoyable in the long term. Consulting with a
healthcare provider or dietitian can help tailor the diet to individual needs
and preferences.

7 Day Meal Plan for SOS-Free combined with Intermittent Fasting

Here's a 7-day meal plan for a Salt, Oil, and Sugar-Free (SOS-Free) diet
combined with intermittent fasting, where meals are eaten at 7 AM and 2
PM. This plan focuses on whole, plant-based foods and avoids added
salt, oil, and sugar.

Day 1

Meal 1 (7 AM):

- Oatmeal made with water, topped with fresh berries and a sprinkle
  of cinnamon.
- A small handful of raw nuts.

Meal 2 (2 PM):

- Quinoa salad with chopped vegetables (cucumber, bell pepper,
  cherry tomatoes), fresh herbs (parsley, mint), and lemon juice.
- Steamed broccoli and carrots.

Day 2

Meal 1 (7 AM):

- Smoothie with spinach, banana, frozen berries, and unsweetened almond milk.
- A small handful of raw sunflower seeds.

Meal 2 (2 PM):

- Lentil stew with tomatoes, carrots, celery, and herbs (oregano, thyme).
- Steamed green beans.

Day 3

Meal 1 (7 AM):

- Chia seed pudding made with unsweetened almond milk and topped with fresh fruit (such as strawberries or blueberries).
- A small handful of raw almonds.

Meal 2 (2 PM):

- Brown rice and black bean bowl with corn, diced tomatoes, cilantro, and lime juice.
- Steamed kale with a splash of apple cider vinegar.

Day 4

Meal 1 (7 AM):

- Whole grain toast with mashed avocado and a sprinkle of red pepper flakes.
- A small apple.

Meal 2 (2 PM):

- Baked sweet potato with a topping of steamed broccoli and a sprinkle of nutritional yeast.

- Mixed greens salad with cherry tomatoes, cucumber, and balsamic vinegar.

Day 5

Meal 1 (7 AM):

- Unsweetened applesauce with a sprinkle of cinnamon and a small handful of walnuts.
- Herbal tea.

Meal 2 (2 PM):

- Chickpea salad with diced cucumber, tomatoes, red onion, and parsley, dressed with lemon juice.
- Steamed cauliflower.

Day 6

Meal 1 (7 AM):

- Fresh fruit salad with a variety of seasonal fruits.
- A small handful of raw pumpkin seeds.

Meal 2 (2 PM):

- Stir-fried vegetables (such as bell peppers, snap peas, carrots, and mushrooms) with tofu, using water for sautéing.
- Brown rice.

Day 7

Meal 1 (7 AM):

- Buckwheat porridge made with water, topped with sliced banana and a sprinkle of chia seeds.
- Herbal tea.

Meal 2 (2 PM):

- Stuffed bell peppers with quinoa, black beans, corn, and diced tomatoes, seasoned with cumin and garlic powder.
- Steamed spinach.

Additional Tips:

1. **Hydration**: Drink plenty of water throughout the day, and consider herbal teas as well.
2. **Herbs and Spices**: Use a variety of herbs and spices to enhance the flavor of your dishes without salt.
3. **Whole Foods**: Focus on whole, unprocessed foods to maintain nutrient density.
4. **Meal Prep**: Prepare larger batches of meals to save time and ensure you stay on track.
5. **Balanced Meals**: Ensure each meal includes a good balance of protein, healthy carbohydrates, and fats from whole food sources.

The Keto Diet Pros and Cons

The ketogenic (keto) diet is a high-fat, low-carbohydrate diet that aims to induce a state of ketosis, where the body burns fat for fuel instead of carbohydrates. Here are the pros and cons of the keto diet, along with an overview of long-term successes and health outcomes.

Pros of the Keto Diet:

1. **Weight Loss**: Many people experience significant weight loss on the keto diet due to reduced appetite and increased fat burning.
2. **Blood Sugar Control**: The diet can improve blood sugar levels and insulin sensitivity, making it beneficial for those with type 2 diabetes.
3. **Improved Mental Clarity**: Some people report better focus and mental clarity on the keto diet, possibly due to the stable energy supply from ketones.
4. **Reduced Inflammation**: The keto diet may reduce inflammation, which is linked to various chronic diseases.
5. **Increased Energy**: Many people find they have more stable and sustained energy levels without the blood sugar spikes and crashes associated with high-carb diets.

Cons of the Keto Diet:

1. **Nutrient Deficiencies**: Restricting carbohydrates can lead to deficiencies in essential nutrients like fiber, vitamins, and minerals found in fruits, vegetables, and grains.
2. **Keto Flu**: Initial side effects can include fatigue, headache, dizziness, nausea, and irritability as the body adjusts to ketosis.

3. **Sustainability**: The restrictive nature of the diet can make it challenging to maintain long-term.
4. **Digestive Issues**: Some people experience constipation or other digestive problems due to low fiber intake.
5. **Risk of Heart Disease**: High intake of saturated fats from animal products can increase the risk of heart disease if not carefully managed.

Long-term Successes and Health Outcomes:

1. **Weight Maintenance**: Some individuals successfully maintain weight loss long-term on a keto diet, particularly if they adopt a balanced approach and include nutrient-dense foods.
2. **Blood Sugar Control**: Long-term adherence can continue to provide benefits for blood sugar control, especially in people with type 2 diabetes or insulin resistance.
3. **Improved Cholesterol Levels**: Some studies show improvements in HDL cholesterol and triglycerides, though LDL cholesterol levels can increase in some individuals.
4. **Reduced Seizures**: The keto diet is well-documented for reducing seizures in people with epilepsy, particularly in children who do not respond to conventional treatments.
5. **Potential Longevity Benefits**: Some research suggests that keto diets may have anti-aging and longevity benefits, although more long-term studies are needed.

Potential Risks:

1. **Cardiovascular Health**: There is concern that high saturated fat intake can negatively impact heart health. It's important to focus on healthy fats like avocados, nuts, seeds, and olive oil.
2. **Bone Health**: Long-term keto dieting may impact bone health, potentially increasing the risk of osteoporosis due to changes in calcium and vitamin D metabolism.
3. **Kidney Health**: The diet can strain the kidneys, particularly in individuals with pre-existing kidney conditions, due to increased protein intake.

4. **Liver Health**: People with liver conditions should be cautious, as the liver is heavily involved in the production of ketones.
5. **Gut Health**: Low fiber intake may negatively affect gut microbiota, which is crucial for overall health.

Conclusion:

The keto diet can offer significant benefits, particularly for weight loss and blood sugar control. However, it's essential to approach it mindfully, ensuring a balanced intake of nutrients and monitoring potential health risks. Consulting with a healthcare provider or dietitian can help tailor the diet to individual needs and ensure it is followed safely and effectively. Long-term studies are still needed to fully understand the health outcomes of sustained keto dieting.

7 Day Meal Plan:

Here's a 7-day meal plan for a keto diet combined with intermittent fasting, where meals are eaten at 7 AM and 2 PM. This plan includes nutrient-dense, keto-friendly meals designed to keep you in ketosis while supporting intermittent fasting.

Day 1

Meal 1 (7 AM):

- Scrambled eggs with spinach and cheese cooked in coconut oil.
- Avocado slices.
- Black coffee or tea.

Meal 2 (2 PM):

- Grilled chicken breast with a side of cauliflower rice.
- Mixed greens salad with olive oil and vinegar dressing.
- A handful of almonds.

Day 2

Meal 1 (7 AM):

- Greek yogurt (full-fat, unsweetened) with a handful of berries and chia seeds.
- Bulletproof coffee (coffee blended with MCT oil and butter).

Meal 2 (2 PM):

- Baked salmon with lemon butter sauce.
- Steamed asparagus.
- Side salad with avocado and olive oil dressing.

Day 3

Meal 1 (7 AM):

- Omelet with mushrooms, bell peppers, and cheese cooked in butter.
- Sliced avocado.
- Herbal tea.

Meal 2 (2 PM):

- Zucchini noodles with pesto sauce and grilled shrimp.
- Side of mixed greens with olive oil and balsamic vinegar.

Day 4

Meal 1 (7 AM):

- Full-fat cottage cheese with a few slices of cucumber and cherry tomatoes.
- Black coffee.

Meal 2 (2 PM):

- Ground beef lettuce wraps with cheese, avocado, and sour cream.
- Roasted Brussels sprouts with olive oil.

Day 5

Meal 1 (7 AM):

- Keto smoothie (spinach, avocado, coconut milk, a scoop of protein powder, and a few berries).
- Herbal tea.

Meal 2 (2 PM):

- Pork chops with garlic butter and steamed broccoli.
- Side salad with mixed greens, feta cheese, and olive oil dressing.

Day 6

Meal 1 (7 AM):

- Chia seed pudding made with coconut milk, topped with a few raspberries and almonds.
- Black coffee.

Meal 2 (2 PM):

- Grilled chicken thighs with a side of sautéed zucchini.
- Greek salad with olives, feta, cucumber, and olive oil dressing.

Day 7

Meal 1 (7 AM):

- Keto pancakes (almond flour-based) with a small amount of sugar-free syrup and butter.
- Bulletproof coffee.

Meal 2 (2 PM):

- Baked cod with a creamy garlic sauce.
- Cauliflower mash with butter.
- Side of steamed green beans.

Additional Tips:

1. **Hydration**: Drink plenty of water throughout the day.
2. **Electrolytes**: Ensure adequate intake of electrolytes, especially during fasting periods.
3. **Healthy Fats**: Include sources of healthy fats such as avocados, olive oil, coconut oil, and fatty fish.
4. **Protein**: Focus on moderate protein intake from high-quality sources.
5. **Vegetables**: Include non-starchy vegetables to provide fiber and essential nutrients.
6. **Snacks**: If needed, keto-friendly snacks like cheese, nuts, or boiled eggs can be included but should be kept to a minimum to maintain the fasting window.

How To Determine Your Ideal Weight- Unraveling The Mystery

Height and weight charts can seem unrealistic because they often don't account for individual variations in body composition, muscle mass, bone density, and other factors that contribute to a person's overall health. These charts typically use a broad, generalized approach to determine an "ideal" weight range based solely on height and sometimes age, without considering these important individual differences.

Why Height and Weight Charts Might Seem Unrealistic:

1. **Individual Variability**: People have different body types (ectomorph, mesomorph, endomorph) which can affect their weight independently of height.
2. **Muscle vs. Fat**: Muscle tissue weighs more than fat tissue. A person with high muscle mass might be classified as overweight or obese by a standard chart despite being healthy and fit.
3. **Bone Density**: Denser bones can contribute to a higher weight, which isn't necessarily a sign of poor health.
4. **Distribution of Weight**: How weight is distributed across the body can impact health more than total weight. For example, central obesity (excess fat around the abdomen) is more strongly associated with health risks than weight distributed evenly.

Determining a Healthy Weight:

1. **Body Composition**: Measure body fat percentage instead of relying solely on weight. This gives a clearer picture of how much of your weight is lean mass versus fat mass.
2. **Waist-to-Hip Ratio**: This ratio can indicate fat distribution and potential health risks associated with central obesity.
3. **Body Mass Index (BMI)**: While it has limitations, BMI can be useful when used in conjunction with other measurements. It's calculated as weight (kg) divided by height (m) squared.
4. **Health Indicators**: Consider overall health markers such as blood pressure, cholesterol levels, blood sugar levels, and overall fitness.
5. **Functional Health**: Evaluate your ability to perform daily activities, physical endurance, and strength. Functional health is often a better indicator of well-being than weight alone.
6. **Consult Health Professionals**: A healthcare provider can assess individual health needs, considering all factors including medical history, lifestyle, and specific health conditions.

Practical Tips:

- Focus on a balanced diet rich in whole foods, lean proteins, healthy fats, and a variety of fruits and vegetables.
- Incorporate regular physical activity, including both aerobic and strength training exercises.
- Monitor your mental and emotional well-being, as stress and mental health can impact physical health.
- Stay hydrated and ensure you're getting enough sleep, both crucial for overall health.

By using a holistic approach that considers multiple factors, you can determine a healthy weight that makes sense for your unique body and lifestyle.

Embracing the Journey: Fasting for a Transformed Life

As we come to the end of our exploration into the world of fasting, I want to leave you with a sense of hope and encouragement. Fasting, in its many forms, has been a profound and transformative experience for many, including myself. Whether you are considering a short-term fast, a cleanse, or a more extended journey, there is something deeply healing and restorative about this practice that touches not just the body, but the mind and spirit as well.

Reflecting on my own journey, I've had the privilege of experiencing various fasting methods firsthand. Juicing for 30 days, embracing the Gerson Therapy (minus the coffee enema), and undertaking a 14-day water-only fast—followed by a thoughtful refeeding period—were some of the most impactful experiences of my life. Each of these methods brought its own unique benefits and challenges. The 14-day water fast, in particular, was perhaps the most profound for my health, offering deep insights and significant changes that were truly life-altering. However, every fasting approach has its own set of pros and cons, and what works best can vary from person to person.

The true beauty of fasting lies in its holistic approach to healing. When done mindfully, fasting can rejuvenate your physical health, sharpen your mental clarity, and deepen your spiritual connection. It's a practice that aligns the body, mind, and spirit, creating a balanced and harmonious state of well-being. Whether you're seeking to cleanse your body, reset your metabolism, or embark on a spiritual journey, fasting offers a powerful tool for transformation.

Remember, the journey of fasting is not a one-size-fits-all endeavor. It's important to approach it with a sense of curiosity and respect for your own body's needs and limitations. There will be challenges along the way, but each challenge is an opportunity for growth and discovery. Embrace the journey with an open heart and a willingness to listen to your body's signals.

As you embark on your own fasting journey, I wish you the very best. May you find clarity, healing, and renewal through your experience. I also want to acknowledge that if you're reading this book, you may be facing mental, physical, or emotional challenges that have led you to explore fasting. It's with this understanding that I want to offer a prayer for you, asking for strength and wisdom as you navigate this path.

A Prayer for Healing and Wisdom

Heavenly Father,

As we conclude this journey through the practice of fasting, I lift up every reader who has ventured into this exploration with a heart full of hope. I ask for Your guidance and blessing as they embark on their own path of fasting, seeking healing and transformation.

Lord, grant them the wisdom to choose the fasting method that best serves their individual needs, and the discernment to listen to their bodies and adjust as necessary. May they experience profound healing and restoration, not just in their physical bodies, but in their minds and spirits as well.

Give them the strength to persevere through the challenges and the grace to embrace the journey with patience and trust. Surround them with Your peace and comfort, and let them feel Your presence in every moment of their fasting experience.

May this practice lead them to greater self-awareness, spiritual growth, and a renewed sense of purpose. Let their fasting journey be a source of profound transformation and a testament to the holistic power of healing.

In Your holy name, we pray,

Amen.

Thank you for joining me on this exploration of fasting. I hope you find
your own path to health and well-being, and that this journey leads you to
a place of balance, clarity, and joy.

Wishing you all the best on your fasting journey.

With warm regards and blessings,

In Health and Faith,

Dr. Jay Korsen